How To Get A Good Night's Sleep

More Than 100 Ways You Can Improve Your Sleep

Richard Graber with Pa

JOHN WILEY & SONS, INC.

New York • Chichester • Weinheim • Brisbane • Singapore • Toronto

The information contained in this book is not intended to serve as
a replacement for professional medical advice. Any use of the
information in this book is at the reader's discretion. The author
and the publisher specifically disclaim any and all liability arising
directly or indirectly from the use or application of any
information contained in this book. A health care professional
should be consulted regarding your specific situation.

ISBN 0-471-34738-8

Printed in the United States of America

10   9   8   7   6   5   4   3   2

Dedication

For Janet, with wide-awake love.

Contents

Chapter 1

Do You Have a Problem?

Strange, but true, it's often difficult to tell if we have a sleep problem. The most obvious result of poor sleep, for whatever reason, is feeling drowsy, lazy, uninspired the next day. No great surprise, right? Except that many of us first notice how dragged out we feel during the day, at work, at play, at anything, before we think of poor sleep.

And there's nothing sacred about the 8 hours a night, except as a rough average of how long most of us sleep. The average now is closer to 7 1/2 hours anyway. So you're not getting your 7 1/2 to 8 hours? It's probably of no consequence unless it's prolonged and you feel sleepy during the day.

We all have occasional nights of poor sleep—not a problem. But several nights in a row of inadequate sleep and we connect the insomnia and the tired daytime feeling. Family physicians know that patients with sleep problems nearly always first complain about tired days.

Another reason it's hard to define sleep problems is the variation among individuals. So most people need the 7 1/2 to 8 hours a night. You may be the one out of ten who needs only 6 hours, or the one out of ten who needs 9 or more.

Famous examples often are used to make a case for those who don't fall within the norms. Einstein needed 10 hours of sleep a night, Churchill got by on 4 and was a master of the catnap.

These days, peer pressures at work (see Chapter 3: Stress in the Marketplace) and in all corners of our lives tend to reward long hours of work, and short hours of sleep. Tell a colleague you need 8 hours of sleep a night and you won't help your image. But get those 8 hours and you will improve your health, your spirits, your energy.

Your need varies somewhat with your emotional state and stress, but your true sleep need does not vary much over longer periods. For example, the total hours you sleep during one week remarkably is within an hour of another week's total, sleep researchers point out.

Remember too, that Grandma was right; some people do need less sleep than others. At least one out of ten adults is a short sleeper.

Also, studies confirm that some of us find it easy to fall asleep at night and stay asleep until morning. Others have trouble falling asleep and staying asleep. We're not identical in our sleep needs. Our needs and sleep habits differ, just as our hat size or height differs. This is not a judgment, merely statistics.

Some of us, I'm told, are alert and ambitious in the morning, while others (I know this second group), find it difficult to get up and get going. Morning people and night people. Grandma talked about them too, and her assertion that "it runs in the family" has truth in it, sleep specialists now admit. It is hereditary to a significant degree. (If you're a morning person married to a night person, it better be true love.)

Many sleep problems are easily corrected, with proper guidance, and you can take charge. With some problems, you'll want medical help, and in a few situations you possibly will need to see a sleep specialist in a sleep clinic. Almost 250 sleep centers across the United States are listed in the Appendix, which starts on page 131. The services are catching up with the need; recent polls show that one in three Americans has sleep problems.

How Much Sleep Do You Need?

Are you getting enough sleep? Think about how you feel during the day. If you spend your days alert, wide awake, and energetic, you're probably getting enough sleep. If not, you probably need to adjust your sleep habits or correct some problems.

If you're uncertain, but feel that you could do fine on less, give it a try. For a week, get to bed a 1/2 hour later than usual, but get up at your regular time. Feel okay? If so, stick with it. Or try

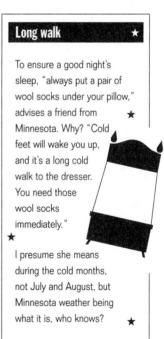

Long walk ★

To ensure a good night's sleep, "always put a pair of wool socks under your pillow," advises a friend from ★ Minnesota. Why? "Cold feet will wake you up, and it's a long cold walk to the dresser. You need those wool socks immediately."
★

I presume she means during the cold months, not July and August, but Minnesota weather being what it is, who knows? ★

adding a 1/2 hour by going to bed earlier if you feel you need more sleep. See what works. There's no danger to this simple trial. One caution: Subtract or add a 1/2 hour at the beginning of your sleep; it's important to keep your time of rising constant.

50 degrees plus ★

In the incomparable book, Home and Health, published in 1879, the authors entitle one section, "Warm or Cold Sleeping-Rooms, Which?" They point out that cold bed-chambers are not advisable and may imperil health. Their advice: "Robust persons may safely sleep in a temperature of forty or under, but the old, the infantile, and the frail, should never sleep in a room . . . under fifty degrees Fahrenheit." ★

You won't catch today's old or infantile or frail sleeping at just over 50 degrees. Folks in 1879 were made of stronger stuff. Or they were cold a lot, which is closer to the truth. ★

★

We recognize sleep problems mainly in retrospect, since we don't even know we're asleep until we wake up. (It's close to the philosophical question about the tree falling in the forest with no one to hear it—does it create sound or not?) And yes, there are times when we awaken at 2 am and come fully awake, unable to return to sleep; we'll get to those wide-awake situations in later chapters.

The National Sleep Foundation, in another approach to assessing your sleep, has issued this brief sleep quotient quiz that calls for yes or no responses:

- Falling asleep is hard for me.

- I have too much on my mind to go to sleep.

- When I wake up during the night, I can't go back to sleep.

- I can't relax because I have too many worries.

- Even when I sleep all night, I still feel tired in the morning.

- I wake up too early.

- Sometimes, I am afraid to close my eyes and go to sleep.

- It takes me more than 30 minutes to fall asleep.

- I am stiff and sore in the morning.

- I feel irritable when I can't sleep.

- I feel that I am dreaming all night long.

Don't think in terms of just last night, but think of your common sleep pattern. If you answered yes to several questions, it is time to take charge and do something about your sleep. There's nothing definitive about that little quiz, but it does point up reasons for thinking about your sleep—and talking with your doctor if you have questions.

Everyone is at risk for poor sleep from time to time, and women a bit more than men. Forty percent or more of women have trouble sleeping, compared with 30 percent of men. The increase is thought due, in part, to women's hormonal shifts that accompany menstruation, pregnancy, and menopause. Changes in progesterone and estrogen levels, for example, can have a sedative effect or bring on uncomfortable effects such as night sweats. Also, some sleep specialists point to the dual roles many women play in bringing home an income and serving as primary caregiver for children or aging parents. (For more on menopause, see *Midlife, Madness, or Menopause: Does Anyone Know What's Normal?* by Patricia J. Richter and Roger Duvivier, MD, Chronimed Publishing, Minneapolis, Minnesota 1995.)

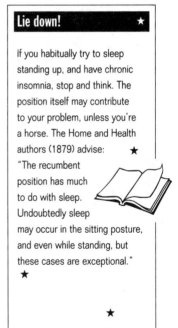

Lie down! ★

If you habitually try to sleep standing up, and have chronic insomnia, stop and think. The position itself may contribute to your problem, unless you're a horse. The Home and Health authors (1879) advise: ★
"The recumbent position has much to do with sleep. Undoubtedly sleep may occur in the sitting posture, and even while standing, but these cases are exceptional." ★

★

Older adults also have frequent sleep problems—as many as half over age 65. Inadequate rest is not an inevitable part of aging, no matter how Grandpa complained when you were a child. The total amount of sleep doesn't change significantly with aging, but the pattern does. Older people tend to get sleepy earlier, wake up more often, and get less "delta" restorative sleep (see Chapter 2: So What is Sleep?), but total sleep, including naps, doesn't vary much.

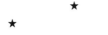
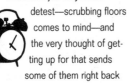

Detestable jobs ★

★

A Pennsylvania woman says, "When I wake up at 3 am, I tell myself to get up and do something constructive, like check the doors and windows. But I'm almost always too tired for all that activity, and fall back asleep." And an Ohio therapist has a nice twist on the "get up and do something" advice. When people complain of nighttime awakenings, she has them think of the household job they most detest—scrubbing floors comes to mind—and the very thought of getting up for that sends some of them right back to sleep. That's what she says.

★

★

★

Sorting Out Insomnia

Classifying insomnia can help you concentrate on what probably is behind your sleep problems. If you remember this one statement, you're ahead of the game: Stress is without question the most common reason for sleeplessness. This includes not only anxiety and feeling uptight, but the regular daily stresses of life that you may have trouble turning off when you go to bed.

Specialists have different classifications of insomnia. One system divides insomniacs into those who can't fall asleep when they go to bed, and those who fall asleep easily enough but cannot stay asleep.

Another way of looking at insomnia is how long it lasts. Transient insomnia lasts 1 to 3 nights, short-term insomnia lasts 3 nights to 3 weeks or so, and chronic insomnia lasts longer than 3 weeks, with no end in sight.

Transient insomnia usually is set off by excitement or stress, sometimes anticipatory. An argument with a loved one can leave your mind churning, but so can a key interview coming up tomorrow. Transient insomnia is more likely when you're traveling. (See Chapter 11: Pursuing Traveling Sleep.)

Short-term insomnia often results from longer stress at work or at home, not necessarily a one-time event.

Chronic insomnia can be the result of an inability to get rid of the shorter forms of insomnia. We sometimes build up worry about our lost sleep and blame ourselves, which leads to more insomnia, which gradually becomes chronic. And of course long-standing tensions—an upsetting marriage, chronic illness in a family member, being stuck in an unproductive, upsetting job—can foster chronic sleeplessness.

On Your Way to Better Sleep

It is often difficult to pinpoint when and why sleep problems occur. Many people ignore or deny the most obvious symptom of sleep problems—drowsiness. Once you do recognize signs of fatigue, the next step is to identify its cause.

We should be so lucky ★

★
I asked a Connecticut writer friend to give me his secrets for marvelous night-after-night sleep, which he claimed to be blessed with. His answer: "My routine is to lie there a few minutes and think of an agenda for the following day, and ZONK, the next thing I know it's 7 in the morning. Not only that, but my wife is even better. She finds it hard to stay awake long enough to get to sleep."

If you're reading this at 2 in the morning, go ahead, say it.

★

Sleep logs are valuable for problem sleepers. A sleep log (as shown in the following sample) is used to record how well you sleep and the factors that can affect sleep. Fill it out for a week or two. Then, look for possible causes of sleeplessness. For instance, it may become clear that an after-dinner drink leads to a restless night. Or, that a 10-minute nap Saturday afternoon recharges your batteries.

If your fatigue persists for more than 2 or 3 weeks, see your doctor or a sleep specialist. A complete medical exam, in conjunction with information from your sleep log, may point to a cause of your sleep problem.

Sleep Log	Mon	Tue
How did you sleep last night?		
What time did you go to bed?		
How long did it take you to fall asleep?		
How many times, and for how long, did you awake during the night?		
What time did you get up?		
Anything unusual about yesterday that affected you?		
Did you consume alcohol/caffeine/nicotine yesterday? What and when?		
Did you take any medications that affect your sleep or wakefulness, such as stimulants or depressants?		
Did you nap yesterday? If so, when and how long?		
Rate last night's sleep overall: good, fair, or poor		

Wed	Thur	Fri	Sat	Sun

The following sleep quiz can be used in conjunction with a sleep log or by itself to zero in on sleep problems.

Sleep Quiz (answer as best you can)

What's your sleep problem? _____

_____

How long has it been going on? _____

_____

What makes it better? _____

_____

What makes it worse? _____

_____

What have you done to remedy the situation? _____

_____

How did it work? _____

_____

What medical problems do you have? _____

_____

What emotional or psychological problems do you have? _____

_____

What medications do you take? _____

_____

Do you smoke? If so, how much? _____

_____

Do you drink? If so, what and how much? _____

_____

Do you take caffeine (cola, coffee, tea, chocolate)? If so, which and how

much? _____

_____

Have you had surgery? What and when? _____

_____

Do you have a chronic medical condition such as diabetes, hyperten-

sion, arthritis? Other? _____

_____

What exercise do you get and how often? _____

_____

Has your diet or weight changed recently? If so, how? _____

_____

Do you have a health complaint as well as your sleep problem? _____

_____

Helpful Categories

You can sort through what may be contributing to your sleep problems by considering these categories:

Emotional problems and lifestyle.
This is the big one, involving more than half of the insomnia, specialists say. See Chapter 5: Depression, Anxiety & Unrest.

Aging and changes in sleep patterns with drops in deep sleep.
See Chapter 4: Sleep Changes with Aging.

Medication and sleeping pills.
Sleeping medication recommendations have changed. See Chapter 10: The Limited Role of Sleeping Pills.

Circadian rhythm upsets.
Night shift work, jet lag, and other problems with your sleep-wake pattern may be at fault. See Chapter 6: Body Clocks Out of Sync.

Chapter 2

So What is Sleep?

Ask a sleep researcher to define sleep and you may get enough explanations to keep you awake all night . . . (but no neat definition; they're still refining it.)

Ask a kindergartner what sleep is and he'll snicker, roll his eyes in disbelief, and say something like, "It's when you lie down and close your eyes and go to sleep. You didn't know that?"

Ask a chronic insomniac, and you may hear, "How should I know? I haven't slept a wink in years."

Only 30 years ago, very little was known about sleep and insomnia, scientifically speaking. Today, that knowledge fills volumes and keeps coming in.

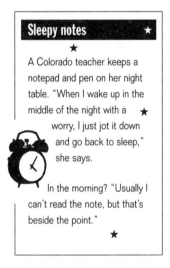

Sleepy notes ★

★

A Colorado teacher keeps a notepad and pen on her night table. "When I wake up in the middle of the night with a ★ worry, I just jot it down and go back to sleep," she says.

In the morning? "Usually I can't read the note, but that's beside the point."

★

For example, a recent review article from *Sleep*, the journal of the American Sleep Disorders Association and Sleep Research Society, is 24 pages long—not unheard of for a scientific paper. Then the author lists his 786 references.

Yes, 786. That's a lot of scientific studies in one field over a couple of decades. Calling this surge an overnight phenomenon is a bad pun but close to the truth. And in many ways it's amazing that we're just now beginning to understand sleep. After all, we spend on average one-third of our lives asleep.

So what have we learned? More important, how will this relatively new knowledge help us sleep better?

Sleep: Dynamic, Restorative

Research has confirmed many age-old ideas about sleep and debunked others. No, sleep is not half way to death. Yes, sleep is restorative (although specialists are still searching for a full explanation for the "recharging" and return of energy.) No, sleep is not a state of total inactivity—a suspension of consciousness.

In fact, sleep is a dynamic behavioral state consisting of a series of cycles, and patterns with a wide range of activity. And we're talking now about normal sleep.

Common sense and direct observation reveal that sleep is not an inert state. "Sleeping like a log" implies a coma-like state, and we've known for years that we do move around in sleep (a sleeping person may make eight to twelve major position shifts per night). Also, we twitch, jerk, mumble or cry out, and in many ways show what seem to be different stages of sleep, from restlessness to being "sound asleep."

Cucumber ice cream ★

★ From Washington state, a middle-aged friend says, "My mother said to keep your feet warm, wear socks to bed and you will sleep. I had no choice. And my grandmother advised that if one has ice cream for dessert at dinner, one does not follow this with acidic food such as cucumbers or oranges, unless one wants to suffer a terrible night of trying to sleep. I have avoided cucumber after dinner ice cream all my life, thus avoiding oh so many terrible sleepless nights." ★

Using electroencephalogram (EEG) tracings of brain waves during sleep, researchers discovered a strong and consistent pattern of sleep cycles. (EEG tracings, indicating the brain's activity, are obtained through harmless electrodes attached to the scalp. The patterns reveal different activities or states, such as awake and alert [alpha waves], deep adult sleep [delta waves], and many more, interpreted by a trained health care provider.) Discovery of REM sleep stages came later and completed the pattern: cycles of light-to-deep sleep followed by rapid eye movement (REM) sleep. Throughout a night of normal sleep, we may go through four to six of these complete cycles.

And this is normal sleep. That is, after a night of many changes in stages and types of sleep, even though we may wake up momentarily many times, we awake refreshed, with the feeling of having slept soundly all night. That is, if all goes well and we get the proper mix of REM and non-REM sleep.

The Components of Sleep

Check the accompanying graph, Normal Adult Sleep Stages. It helps to visualize the pattern. Note the "skyline" look to the graph. Sleep specialists call it sleep architecture—the arrangement of sleep components.

Normal Adult Sleep Stages

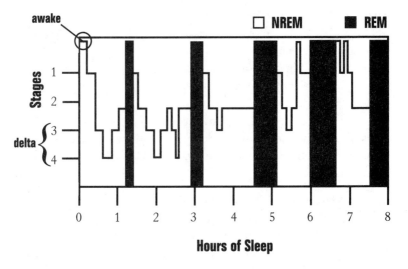

Note the change in proportions of sleep types. Early, deep delta sleep predominates. Later, delta fades as REM duration rises.

There are two basic types of sleep—REM and non-REM. In REM sleep, our eyes move rapidly behind closed lids as we look around in our sleep and dreams. Non-REM sleep is a term for all the rest—what might be thought of as conventional sleep. But non-REM itself consists of different stages.

Here are the changing cycles during normal sleep:

- Awake, you relax, lie down and close your eyes, waiting for sleep. You cannot will it to come; you need to relax and accept it. Your muscle tone is still high, your eyes may still move, and the EEG shows low-voltage alpha waves, as during relaxed wakefulness. Say you go to bed at 10 pm. It should take you no more than a few minutes to a half hour to fall asleep.

- You enter Stage 1 sleep for a few seconds to as long as 10 minutes. Stage 1 is a light, almost twilight zone sleep. It's easy to be aroused in Stage 1, and if this happens, you may not even remember being asleep. Your muscles relax and your pulse and breathing become more shallow and regular. The EEG shows mixed low-voltage waves. Say you fall asleep at 10:10 and complete Stage 1 at 10:15.

- You enter Stage 2 for 30 to 45 minutes. Stage 2 is a little deeper sleep. This is the first real sleep stage—that is, you are not at all aware of your surroundings, your breathing further diminishes, and even if someone lifted your eyelids, sleep specialists point out, you would not see. (Undoubtedly true, and they have lifted an eyelid or two. If someone were to lift mine, I believe I would wake up and then see, but the point is moot. We're not going to try.) Although nearly half of your night will be spent in Stage 2 on average, less is known about this stage than any other. The EEG shows groups of regular fast waves (sleep spindles) and spiking waves. Say you sleep in Stage 2 from 10:15 to 11.

- You enter Stages 3 and 4 for 40 to 70 minutes, longer during the first hour or two of sleep, and decreasing dramatically in the cycles toward the end of the night. Some sleep specialists lump Stage 3 and Stage 4 as deep or delta sleep, characterized on EEG tracings by the slow delta waves—over 20 percent in Stage 3 deepening to 50 percent or more in Stage 4. Your sleep changes are gradual and this is your deepest

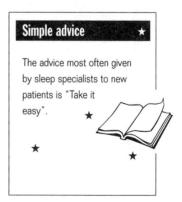

Simple advice ★

The advice most often given by sleep specialists to new patients is "Take it easy".

sleep, the most restorative physically, and the closest we come to hibernating. Say you complete delta sleep at 12.

- REM sleep comes at the end of your first sleep cycle. However, you may leave delta sleep as you entered it, only reversed. You move quickly back from Stage 4 to 3 to 2 to 1, then into REM sleep, rather than waking up. REM sleep appears closest to being awake, with similar EEG tracings and dramatically increased cerebral activity. The first REM period lasts a few minutes, in each succeeding cycle it lasts longer, and the final one may last up to an hour or more.

You slip from one stage of sleep to another without being aware of it or showing outward signs, except for REM. A full sleep cycle consists of the four non-REM Stages and REM. During a normal night's sleep, you may go through four to six cycles, depending on how long you sleep. Notice how the proportion of different types of sleep changes with each cycle. As you continue through the night, delta sleep diminishes to almost nothing, and REM sleep increases.

As we age, (see Lifetime Sleep Patterns, page 32), the proportion of delta sleep fades, although other stages, including REM, remain constant.

The EEG or brain wave tracings show characteristic patterns that help sleep specialists tell one stage from another. If your main interest is good sleep, don't worry about them. If you're curious, for more detail see the suggested reading list on page 130.

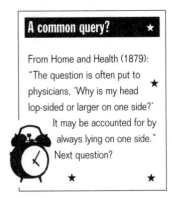

A common query? ★

From Home and Health (1879):
"The question is often put to physicians, 'Why is my head lop-sided or larger on one side?' It may be accounted for by always lying on one side."
Next question?

★ ★

More on REM Sleep

You normally enter your first REM sleep about 90 minutes after first falling asleep. As noted, the first episode of REM is short, completing the first sleep cycle, and it increases with each additional cycle. The last REM phase usually is at least half an hour and occasionally an hour or more.

Unlike delta sleep, with its controlled slow metabolism, REM sleep is active. Yes, you remain asleep, but pulse, temperature, blood pressure, and respiration change.

During REM, women have clitoral engorgement and men usually get penile erections (one way physicians check for physiological impotence). The erections have no apparent connection with sensual content of dreams. Young men have four or five a night, while men in their 70s have two or three, on average.

At the end of the REM sleep phases, you may awaken for a moment and go back to sleep without being aware of it.

With all the activity during REM sleep, think of it as a phase when your brain wakes up but you do not. During delta sleep, blood is concentrated elsewhere with relatively little going to the brain. During REM, blood supply to the brain increases as it becomes more active.

Sleep specialists generally agree that during REM, your brain is hard at work; it may be sorting, working, dreaming. Restoration of your emotional self seems to take place in REM sleep, the way physical restoration takes place during delta sleep. If you miss REM sleep, you may find it more difficult to understand and deal with your life happenings.

Most dreams and certainly the most intense dreams occur during REM sleep. The movement of your eyeballs behind closed lids may result from your looking at what's happening in those dreams.

The intense dreams may raise your heart rate dramatically, and result in twitching muscles. This may be like your dog when he twitches his paws in sleep and you think he's after a rabbit in his dreams. If you were awake, you would shout and run away from danger. In sleep, your muscles are partially paralyzed.

By the way, it would seem that a person in REM sleep would be easily aroused, given the erratic and active nature of the sleep, but not so. Some specialists refer to REM as paradoxical sleep for this reason. It's light sleep in some ways, including EEG tracings, but deep sleep in others.

Pew potato ★

An old Minnesota friend was forced as a child to attend ★ church services every Sunday. Back then, the sermon was delivered in Norwegian, which his parents understood, but he did not. Consequently, he slept during the sermon. ★

To this day—long past child-hood—he immediately falls asleep whenever he attends church, and yawns even when walking by a church. His faith is solid. It works every time.

★

★

More happenings during sleep: These days, sleep specialists are able to monitor far more than just your brain waves on EEG. Sleep centers are set up to keep track of a variety of functions as you sleep through the night, all recorded as waves on a wide continuous sheet of EEG paper.

The patient sleeps in a room usually resembling a bedroom, while technicians receive the signals on a polysomnograph in a nearby room. In addition to electrodes glued to the scalp for EEG brain wave tracings, a patient may be hooked up with electrodes (small flat painless discs) to the legs to record any twitching, to the temples to record eye movement, to the chin to record muscle tension, and on the chest to measure heart function. Sensors in front of the nose can record breathing temperature and airflow. Bands around the abdomen and chest record breathing movement.

Remarkably, with all of these hookups and sometimes more, patients do sleep during their night at a sleep lab. Sometimes patients sleep very well, waking up refreshed and a little embarrassed at not having come up with findings to back their complaints of insomnia. What this suggests to sleep specialists is that their problems are caused by something at home, something to do with their routines.

Chapter 3

Stress in the Marketplace

Susan is a highly motivated 35-year-old state lobbyist for an environmental group. She spends more time in the Statehouse than in her own office. In a way, Susan is a portable office.

She sets up in the Statehouse lobby, surrounded by her laptop computer (loaded with tons of data on environmental issues) and her beeper so she's constantly available to legislators and clients, her cellular phone, legislative reference books, copies of bills, bags full of jelly beans, an apple, and bottles of soda water.

Recognize her? Her sleep is shot, she admits.

Bert is a 47-year-old farmer, up at 5 am on a spring day after a week of rainy days. He checks his computer's radar weather report, anxious to get seed in the ground. It looks promising. He fills the seed bins on his enormous planter, settles into his field work, and has 160 acres of his 2,800-acre farm planted with corn by noon.

With his investment in machinery, seed, insurance, and all the trappings of a modern Midwest farm business, Bert starts most mornings at his computerized office. He checks market prices by computer as he drives his enclosed tractor, winds up his days in the office, logging his progress, figuring his chances, accessing his databases. Bert has troubled sleep and a troubled stomach. He's down in the dumps too often and drags through the days.

When Sleep Suffers

Back to basics. In the 19th century, people in this country slept an average of 9 1/2 hours a night. In those pre-light bulb, pre-electricity days, there wasn't that much to do in the evening. And our ancestors had put in long hours of hard physical work, so when darkness came, they were ready for bed. Also, they had no faxes to be answered, no cellular phones or e-mail to interrupt things, no Internet to play with, no all-night television.

By the 1950s and 1960s, we slept an average of 7 to 8 hours a night, and today it's closer to 7.

Why? We react to the increasing complexity of our days, days filled with pressures and stress, and the first thing to go is sleep. Today, if you get by on short hours of sleep, it's often considered dynamic, a take-charge approach to work and life. If you admit that you really need 8 to 9 hours of sleep, too often folks may think you lack drive.

But, it's common sense to get the sleep you need. Inadequate sleep leaves you with battered nerves, lapses in memory, mood swings, irritability—and more inadequate sleep. Sooner or later, job performance will suffer too.

Consider: Far and away the most common reason for sleeplessness is stress—not necessarily momentous stress, but the usual stresses of life. A tight schedule with no time for inviting good sleep leaves us thinking about those stresses at night, not being able to turn them off. Probably the most common advice sleep specialists give to patients they see is "Relax. You're trying too hard."

> **The writing life . . .** ★
>
> ★
> "It's getting worse, this time thing. Our entire society is hooked up to beepers, cellular phones, answering machines and services, faxes, and computerized appointment calendars. ★
> We are expected to be productive every waking moment, and get by on little sleep. Everyone works overtime and in addition to that, we have to eat fiber, exercise, meditate, volunteer, and make sure our kids get in the gifted program." ★
>
> From "How to Make Time to Write," by Robyn Carr, June 1995, Writer's Digest magazine, used with permission.
>
> ★

Stress: More than Meets the Eye

It's easy to blame stress and today's fast pace for insomnia and any other problem we come up with, but more important is how we react. Stress has taken a bad rap. In the face of widespread media reports of the perils of stress, we need to remember that stress is a common and necessary part of living. No stress, no life.

Hans Selye, the Austrian endocrinologist who spent more than 50 years studying stress (some of us think he invented it), says death is the only stress-free state.

Stress comes in an infinite variety, not just from cataclysmic events such as war, pestilence, flood, or famine. Recent studies emphasize that what really gets to us more often is the common irritant. We are much more likely to become stressed out and lose sleep over the hassles; they wear away if we let them.

Remember these two rules of stress management:

Rule 1

Don't sweat the small stuff.

Rule 2

It's all small stuff.

Does that seem flip? Maybe, but it works when we can adhere to it. And it makes sense when we realize what causes stressful situations.

Most of us are stressed by family concerns such as marriage problems, quarrels between parents and kids, teenage rebellion, divorce and the problems that often follow, and the like. Family stress can include the birth of your first grandchild too, or a happy wedding of your son or daughter. Not all stress is negative.

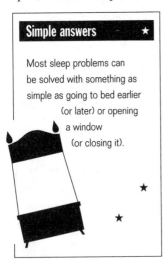

Simple answers

Most sleep problems can be solved with something as simple as going to bed earlier (or later) or opening a window (or closing it).

Then there's your job. It's realistic to feel some stress over job longevity in today's business world, as well as bosses you know can't do their work, co-workers who try to upstage you at every opportunity, pension plans that collapse with no explanation, and other worries.

The state of our health may produce

stress. If you have a minor operation scheduled, yes, it makes sense to be concerned about it, but do not let yourself become stressed out. If you are overweight, get no exercise, and eat a grand array of things you know aren't good for you, that can be stressful. And most of us have been there.

Other stressors can be anything from your neighbor's rock band rehearsing, to lining up a date, to rude people stepping ahead of you in the movie ticket line. (Yes, it's almost a stereotype, but that doesn't help.)

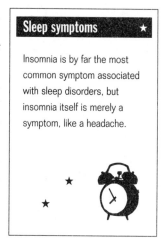

Sleep symptoms ★

Insomnia is by far the most common symptom associated with sleep disorders, but insomnia itself is merely a symptom, like a headache.

And let's not forget a sudden rainstorm when you're about to drive to the airport to pick up your spouse. Or the neighbor's dog squatting directly over your newly seeded lawn. Or the concert tickets you can't find and time's running out. You know your stress points. Recognize them for what they are—the hot button stimuli that may set you off.

And the Reaction?

Just as important as the outside stresses—more important, many specialists feel—is how we react to them. It's one thing to recognize a stressful situation, and another to cool it.

Most of us know the fight-or-flight phenomenon—a holdover from primitive days that's still working, but in bizarre ways. Okay, when stress hits, our body pours adrenalin into the bloodstream, blood pressure rises, heart pounds, mouth goes dry, arteries narrow, pupils dilate, and so on.

Eons ago, the changes may have been for immediate survival. With a saber-toothed tiger about to pounce, the fast pulse and more blood to the muscles gave us maximum speed. Since we had little chance of outdoing the tiger, we needed help for a speedy escape.

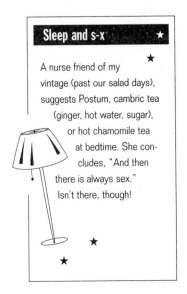

Sleep and s-x ★

★

A nurse friend of my vintage (past our salad days), suggests Postum, cambric tea (ginger, hot water, sugar), or hot chamomile tea at bedtime. She concludes, "And then there is always sex." Isn't there, though!

★

★

Today, the stressor may be your boss, who has no intention of eating you, but asks for the third night in a row if you won't please work overtime so said boss can entertain out of town customers. If your blood pressure goes ballistic, you feel physiologically fit and ready to toss him or her out of the 42nd floor window. You can't do it. Society frowns on it. So you learn to live with it.

But not all of us learn to live with it well, and our sleep suffers. Lack of sleep leaves us ragged the next day, and the tension-insomnia combination becomes self-perpetuating.

Sleep specialists know the high achiever who races through the workday, works late, gets home at 8:30, hits the park trail for a 5-mile run, showers, gulps down dinner, checks briefly on family if there is one, checks e-mail, etc., vaults into bed at 11 and demands sleep. Only it doesn't work.

You may be able to run other portions of your life on a tight schedule, but there is no way you can will yourself to sleep. You need to relax enough for sleep to come to you.

What Course to Take

We all experience minor stresses each day, and feel none the worse. But a series of stressful situations or a series of overreactions, should make us take a hard look at what's going on.

The Surgeon General's office advises that excessive stress may have serious implications for physical and mental health. It contributes to gastrointestinal disorders such as ulcers, cardiovascular disorders like hypertension, respiratory disorders like allergies, musculoskeletal disorders such as arthritis and low back pain, and inhibition of the immune system.

How to hold down that level of stress reaction? One unlikely self-help technique is a positive, active attitude. Hans Selye has said with certainty, "Nothing erases unpleasant thoughts more effectively than concentration on pleasant ones."

Laugh your cares away? I too thought it was too good to be true and too simplistic to be effective, but I have changed my mind. Humor is indeed one way of relieving or reducing stress.

I learned this from Dale L. Anderson, MD, a remarkable doctor and Mayo Clinic trained surgeon who no longer practices surgery. Now he is director of Complementary Medicine at the highly regarded Park Nicollet Clinic in Minneapolis, and is a nationally recognized speaker on healing and humor in health.

Dr. Anderson, an MD for nearly 40 years, had severe burns on his hands and face from a childhood accident. Years later, he had to admit that his hands weren't up to his rigorous practice of surgery, and he had to make a career change. His interest led him to studies in pain treatment and mobilization techniques and ways of dealing with stress.

"Laughter raises your inner uppers," Dr. Anderson says, referring to the endorphins, the body's natural tranquilizers. "When you laugh, your body produces endorphins, the chemicals that have a calming effect in people who are stressed. Next time you feel tense, look in the mirror and have a good belly laugh."

And if you don't feel like laughing or cannot laugh on command?

"Fake it," he says. "Go ahead. Soon you'll be chuckling, smiling, grinning. You don't need to laugh 'til you leak, but a few chuckles every day will be beneficial."

As an aging, strictly amateur Dixie clarinetist, I love that command. You say you can't do it? Fake it. That's going to work for laughing as it works for jazz.

A long sleep ★

Those of us who live to be one hundred will have spent some 30 years asleep. From that ★ perspective, it makes sense to try for the best, most pleasant sleep possible.

★

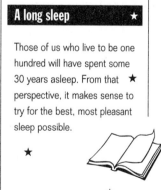

★

Also, during periods of feeling stressed, build laughter and good feeling into your day, he advises. Try to be around people you enjoy and, as much as possible, steer clear of those you find emotionally draining.

Talk Your Way Through

How often do you talk to yourself? Probably more often than you realize, and Dr. Anderson suggests you take advantage of this. Talk positively to yourself, not negatively.

It's a simple concept that may work wonders for you in times of stress.

"Have you ever watched children tying their shoes?" Dr. Anderson asks. "If they're just learning, they talk themselves through it, which makes it so much easier. This self-talk can benefit adults too, especially when they switch from negative to positive talk.

"Watch for the negative response to situations, such as 'I shouldn't have done that,' 'I'll never make it to the meeting on time' or 'This job is awful.'"

He calls it "negative chatter."

"Negative thoughts create tension," he says. "So make a conscious effort to respond positively to stressful situations. Watch out for the won'ts and shouldn'ts. Think and talk to yourself positively. 'It won't be easy, but I can do this again and make it better.' 'I'll do as much of this as I can.' Encourage yourself."

Chapter 4

Sleep Changes with Aging

When Grandma nods off for a daytime nap, don't be too critical . . . unless she's driving a bus at the time. Innocent naps are part of the changing pattern of sleep with age. (Studies suggest that our bodies may be set up for one afternoon nap a day; often it's the older folks who can take advantage of this, although too many or too long naps can disrupt nighttime sleeping.)

The sleep changes in general are no more serious than changes in hair color or vision as we age, and the changes differ widely among individuals. On average, as you move through middle age and into old age, you can expect a different pattern of sleep, but not much change in the amount of sleep you need.

It's important to know what to expect. It is not normal to have continuing trouble falling asleep at night and it is not normal to fall asleep frequently during the day.

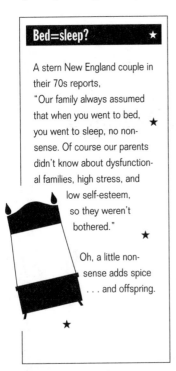

Bed=sleep? ★

A stern New England couple in their 70s reports,
"Our family always assumed that when you went to bed, ★ you went to sleep, no nonsense. Of course our parents didn't know about dysfunctional families, high stress, and low self-esteem, so they weren't bothered." ★

Oh, a little nonsense adds spice . . . and offspring.

As we age, our bodies become less efficient at sustaining sleep. Our sleep becomes shallow and more fragile, with shorter sleep periods that are much more easily disrupted. Keep in mind that the changes in sleep patterns with age are dramatic in some people, subtle in others, and almost nonexistent in a very few.

Age-related changes sometimes mask sleep disorders that increase as we get older, so it's important to look for causes of insomnia and not just chalk it up to increased age.

Early in life, most of us tend to fall asleep quickly and sleep soundly. As we age, we tend to find it more difficult settling down to sleep, we awaken more often at night, and we take longer to get back to sleep. "Old" and "aging" are relative terms, but many of us notice changes in sleep patterns from about age 35 on, and more certainly in our 50s and 60s.

So our sleep tends to be more fragile—less time in the deep restorative sleep, and more time in shallower sleep stages which means we are more likely to be aroused by noises, movement, and the like. Studies show that the daily total sleep declines from 7-plus hours in early adulthood to 7 by age 60 and 6 by age 70. Remember, these are averages.

As for the widespread belief that older people need less sleep, it's not that simple. Our bodies may become less successful at retaining sleep as we age, we may find it easier to nap during the day, and we may awaken much more frequently during the night. Some people from about age 60 and older awaken briefly at least 150 times a night. Small wonder such sleep is described as fragile.

All those awakenings have little to do with how we feel in the morning. Some older people are aware of these brief moments of wakefulness (up to 15 seconds, on average) and feel that they have been awake all night. Others don't notice, and usually report sound sleep. By comparison, young adults awaken briefly only five times a night or so. The difference may be a direct result of the time spent in deep delta sleep—much more in the younger, much less in the older sleepers. Both ages spend about the same proportion of sleep time in REM sleep, the active dreaming stage.

True north ★

In 1879, the authors of Home and Health advised as follows: "Sleeping rooms (they didn't call them bedrooms then) should always be so arranged, if possible, as to allow the head of the sleeper to be ★ turned toward the north. Frequently, in cases of sickness, a person will find it impossible to obtain rest if his head is in any other direction, and often a cure is retarded for a long time. This arrangement puts the sleeper in harmony with the electrical currents caused by the motion of the earth on its axis. Try this and see." ★

Ridiculous? Maybe, but as the authors suggest, why not give it a try? What's to lose? Except that today, so few of us know which way is north.

★

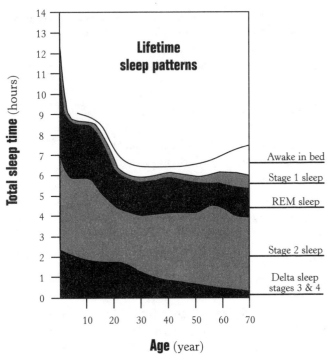

Delta sleep decreases markedly with age, while REM and Stage 2 remain quite constant.

As we pass from age 30 through age 60, most of us notice that we sleep less soundly, which is normal. In our 20s, deep sleep may be reduced by almost half, in middle age (30 to 60) our sleep becomes noticeably more shallow. By age 40, Stage 4 sleep essentially disappears, and as we age further, we tend to lose more of our Stage 3 sleep. On average, we are three times more likely to have nighttime awakenings at age 60 than at age 20. Age 60 and older, most people awaken at least once a night to go to the bathroom.

Younger than age 40, healthy people spend just 1 to 2 percent of bedtime awake. By age 70, a healthy person will spend 12 to 15 percent of time in bed awake.

What Affects Sleep in Older Adults?

Think of the causes of insomnia in middle age and beyond in four categories: (1) medical problems, (2) primary sleep disorders, (3) medications, or (4) lifestyle. These interferences with sleep occur at any age, but are more likely to affect sleep in middle and old age.

As we age and our sleep becomes less restorative on average, other factors also become increasingly important. A National Institutes of Health panel of experts reported in 1990 that more than half of people age 65 or over have disturbed sleep, and insomnia is by far the most common complaint that brings them to the doctor's office (with the possible exception of upper respiratory infections.)

Medical Problems

We all have medical problems from time to time, but as we move through middle age toward old age, we're apt to have more—and more chronic conditions.

Asthma, bronchitis, emphysema and other respiratory disorders can interrupt breathing at night, leading to poor sleep.

Pain and stiffness from arthritis, other rheumatic problems, and fibrositis (muscle tenderness) can interrupt sleep many times. Muscle pain and stiffness from any cause make it almost impossible to move in bed without waking yourself up.

Itching and allergic reactions can interfere with sleep at any age, but particularly in middle age and beyond. Note: Body chemistry changes with age, and allergic reactions may also change. My grandfather, who spent all his life in outdoor work, was immune to poison ivy—could walk through fields of it with no effect, and took modest pride in this . . . until he was 80 years old. Then he came down

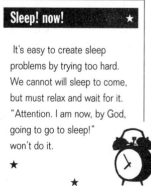

Sleep! now! ★

It's easy to create sleep problems by trying too hard. We cannot will sleep to come, but must relax and wait for it. "Attention. I am now, by God, going to go to sleep!" won't do it.

★

★

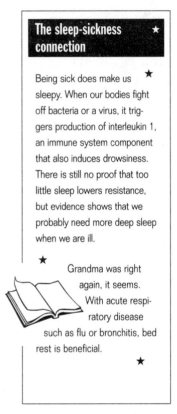

The sleep-sickness ★ connection

Being sick does make us ★ sleepy. When our bodies fight off bacteria or a virus, it triggers production of interleukin 1, an immune system component that also induces drowsiness. There is still no proof that too little sleep lowers resistance, but evidence shows that we probably need more deep sleep when we are ill.

★ Grandma was right again, it seems. With acute respiratory disease such as flu or bronchitis, bed rest is beneficial. ★

with his first poison ivy reaction, which was a rouser.

The pain of an angina attack at night rouses people. These attacks—when the heart doesn't receive enough oxygen—often occur during REM sleep. Hypertension, coronary artery disease, and peripheral vascular disease all can contribute to insomnia.

Any skeletal problem such as osteoporosis can interfere with sleep because of the pain associated.

Heartburn is a common sleep preventer. It's an acid reflux when stomach acids back up into the esophagus. If you tend to have heartburn, you know it is more likely when you lie down, so raising the head of the bed is one way to correct it—as well as modifying your diet.

Other problems that can interfere with sleep, perhaps less directly, are diabetes, hyperthyroidism, and other endocrine disorders, and uremia and other kidney problems.

If your sleep is disturbed by a medical problem, or you think it may be, the solution lies with correcting the problem, not just the insomnia. Often, a thorough physical examination is in order, so consult your physician. Even with a chronic condition or a recurrent condition (diabetes, arthritis, dermatitis, as examples), a change may precipitate sleep problems. Be sure to consult your doctor on a regular basis to avoid such problems as much as possible.

Primary Sleep Disorders

Most of these conditions also can happen at any age, but are more common as we age. See Chapter 12 for details on sleep apnea, narcolepsy, periodic limb movements, restless leg syndrome, advance sleep phase syndrome (too early to bed, too early rising), and the parasomnias.

Pharmacologic Problems

Overuse of prescription and nonprescription drugs to aid sleep is most common in the elderly. People over age 65 make up 13 percent of the American population, but take more than 30 percent of prescription drugs and 40 percent of all sleeping pills.

From about age 40 on, the rate of metabolizing medications slows down. What used to be an adequate dose of a medication can be an overdose as you age. With slower metabolism, the drug stays in your body longer. A medication that works to help you sleep at 40, may keep you sedated the next day at 50.

Pills of any kind that caused mild insomnia at age 30, can cause severe insomnia when you're 60 or 70. Be sure to check with your doctor before taking medications, and check promptly if you experience bothersome side effects as you age. Often, a simple medication adjustment can work wonders with sleep problems in middle age and beyond.

It pays to check with your doctor especially if you take any of these insomnia-producing drugs:

- some drugs for high blood pressure
- drugs with amphetamine
- drugs with caffeine
- steroid preparations
- some antidepressants
- some thyroid preparations

- bronchodilating drugs for asthma or chronic obstructive lung disease
- sleeping pills and tranquilizers (apt to bring insomnia on the nights you don't take them)
- adrenocorticotropic hormone (ACTH)
- drugs for Parkinsonism
- nasal decongestants
- some cancer medications.

Be sure your doctor knows all the drugs you're taking, including the nonprescription medications. For your own information, and to help your doctor give you the best care, keep a log of medications. Almost inevitably, we take a few more as we age. Don't lose track. Jot down the medication, who prescribed it, when, and when you stopped taking it and why. Also, chart any changes in dosage. This helps with the simple changes that may help you immediately—taking some medications at night rather than during the day, reducing the dose, or substituting a different drug for the same condition. Do this for your nonprescription drugs too.

Caffeine, of course, is a drug, but so many of us drink coffee, tea, hot chocolate, soft drinks without thinking about the caffeine load we're taking on, that it bears special emphasis. (See Chapter 7: How's Your Sleep Hygiene?)

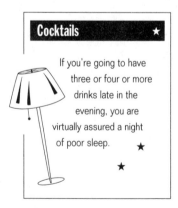

Cocktails ★

If you're going to have three or four or more drinks late in the evening, you are virtually assured a night of poor sleep. ★

★

We may toss off cups of coffee or tea throughout the day and evening without a care, but as you know, our body and brain are well aware of the caffeine effect. We differ widely in our reaction to caffeine, but in general, keep your intake down to 250 to 300 milligrams a day or you'll nearly always have insomnia that night. That's two or three cups maximum all day. (If you must drink them, do it in the morning.) With increasing age, it often takes far less to produce insomnia. The smart thing to do: give up caffeine entirely.

And alcohol. A glass or two of wine at dinner is fine. More than that, especially any drink in the evening, may help you get to sleep but to your regret when you wake a few hours later. That rebound effect is more pronounced in elderly people.

Lifestyle

The stereotypical view of middle age and old age as a time of slowing down, dragging around, sitting alone at home and wondering why the kids or grandchildren never call has little relevance these days. Surely there are older people who fit the stereotype, but it's a small percentage of the middle age and older crowd.

As we move through our 40s and 50s into the "retirement years," how do we affect our sleep and vice versa? Generally, a lot is going on. We have a greater incidence of specific sleep disorders. We have apnea, advanced sleep phase syndrome, periodic limb movements, restless leg syndrome, REM sleep behavior disorder (when we act out our dreams, crash into lamps, fall out of bed, totter down the stairs) . . . it's a far cry from the traditional notion of sleep time as a period of quiet and rest.

> ### Great Catherine ★
>
> Catherine the Great (1729- ★ 1796), empress of Russia, advocated sex six times a day, and took her own advice. As a young ruler, she had 21 official lovers on call, later beefed up to 80. Why her insatiable appetite? She suffered from insomnia, and claimed that sexual congress was the best sleeping tonic. No one argued the point.
>
> ★
>
> ★

Not that many people will pile up all those sleep disturbances and more, but the lifestyle of middle age and older does include a lot of possibilities. The REM sleep disorder, for example, usually happens in men older than 50. In normal sleep, the body is effectively paralyzed during REM sleep, allowing for just twitches. Not so with REM sleep disorder, which removes some of the body's restraints and lets the people act out their dreams with forceful behavior. The medication clonazepam helps improve sleep and control the dream-related physical action. (See Chapter 12 for more on primary sleep disorders.)

Some habits of middle and old age persons lead to certain sleep problems, but at the same time, modification of these behaviors often brings relief. Those of us who looked forward to times when the kids were on their own and the mortgage was paid have had some surprises in recent years. The tranquility (?) of retirement has left some people hanging on the ropes. The major investment in college tuitions, the absence of jobs for our college graduates, the return home of our college graduates, the vanishing of our own job security, the mixed blessings of early retirement . . . fill in your own list.

Also, with age we become more familiar with loss of loved ones, friends, cherished authors, favorite entertainers ("What do you mean, you've never heard of Ernie Kovacs?").

It's all too easy to slip into overwhelming longing for the good old days and the rose-colored glasses times of our youth. Too many of us become boring reciters of how great times past were—neglecting to remember that when we were young, we found this line of talk utterly boring.

Some pleasant thoughts about times past are fine, and predictable, but fixation on the good old days and the lousy hand you've been dealt for your old age can be harmful to your health. And to your sleep.

Insomnia increases with age, especially among those retired people who do not lead an active life. What may begin as feeling blue has a way of becoming chronic in some older people. The prototype of an aged insomniac may be the retired person who gets up late because it's allowed now, sits around the house because he or she doesn't have to go to work, watches television or something equally innocuous, eats erratically, takes frequent naps because no one says No, and is surprised he or she has a hard time getting to sleep and staying asleep.

The progress of depression may be gradual, and linked with sleep deprivation. Sometimes a situation can set off a period of feeling blue—

loss of a friend, bills piling up, hospitalization. The blues can stay with you if you focus on your poor sleep with the early arousal, typical of sleeping pill or alcohol rebound. Early arousal, of course, may also be a sign of depression.

If you think you may be depressed, see if you have other indications—loss of energy, loss of appetite, loss of weight, loss of interest in sex, feelings of hopelessness, guilt. And see your doctor. Depression or any other condition in the elderly can and should be treated, rather than passed off as part of getting old. Same with your insomnia.

Often, the causes of depression-related sleep problems are insufficient physical or mental activity—a bit like trying to fall asleep when you're not tired. And anxieties. One anxiety more common in the elderly is a fear of letting go, which is linked to the fear of death. For some, this fear makes it difficult to relax and fall asleep, and counseling may be the key.

> ### Gatsby awake ★
>
> Novelist F. Scott Fitzgerald, one of the truly great insomniacs, offered two quotations that reveal his frame of mind: "An Egyptian proverb says ★ one of the worst things is to be in bed and sleep not." And "In a real dark night of the soul it is always three o'clock in the morning." Fitzgerald lived his life in double-time and died at age 44. His career is a classic object lesson in how to guarantee debilitating insomnia.
>
>

Some sleep problems in the elderly are expected and easily handled. For example, the advanced sleep-phase syndrome (too early to bed, too early to rise) is common, generally from the lack of deep restorative sleep. Many adapt, but many find their bodies are ready for bed earlier than they want, often well before 9 pm. This means early awakening, and it can be frustrating to be awake early when others are sleeping and be sleepy in the evening when others are socially active.

Often, moving the bedtime back to 11 pm or midnight seems as though it should work and allow for later arising, but the body's internal clock doesn't often agree, and elderly people still wake up early. One solution is chronotherapy, involving a series of prescribed bed-

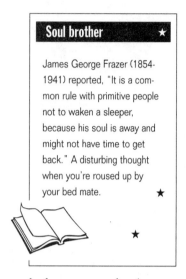

Soul brother ★

James George Frazer (1854-1941) reported, "It is a common rule with primitive people not to waken a sleeper, because his soul is away and might not have time to get back." A disturbing thought when you're roused up by your bed mate. ★

★

times that move backward around the clock—say in 3-hour jumps every 2 days—until you reach the desired bedtime. After reaching this, keep your bedtime hour regular. (More about chronotherapy on page 55.)

Scheduling is a key to better health, better outlook, better sleep among the elderly. With new freedom, the tendency is to stay in bed late, nap when you wish, eat when you wish, and take advantage of your freedom.

Enjoy yourself but don't abandon routines, say sleep specialists. Get out of bed at your regular time, meet friends and get out of the house at regular times, have your meals at regular times—and don't forget the soothing routines such as a hot soak before bed, massaging those tired muscles, and all your sleep hygiene routines (including sex).

Sundowning

Sundowning, sometimes called nocturnal wandering, is frequent in some old people, especially those with mild senile dementia or those who have had a stroke. As we age, some of us need more stimulation to keep steady, to keep oriented to our surroundings and functioning as we want to. At some point, our aging brains enable us to do this during the day, but at sundown, with decreased stimulation, we find it difficult to remain oriented. We can easily become agitated or confused.

This is sundowning, or the sundowner's syndrome. It's easy to accept stimulation during the day when we don't even think about it—the look of our living quarters, the meals on a regular schedule, activities to take care of, interaction with other people. But with dusk, especially for those of us living alone, so many of these cues are removed. It's a delicious time of the day, as one writer says, but not if you're a sundowner.

There is no single treatment for sundowner's syndrome, and the situation needs to be addressed in a common-sense way. If you, or someone you know, are bothered by this disorientation near dusk, try to arrange for someone to be with you during that time, and preferably all night. Turn on the lights, play some familiar music, do familiar things with your friend or spouse, and don't worry if you're a little afraid of the dark; it's to be expected at some stage.

It's important to protect yourself, or your sundowning friend, because the condition can lead to nocturnal wandering. Try to surround yourself with a few people close to you, with pleasant and bright activities, and an evening routine that reminds you of your orientation—where you are and what time it is.

If you suspect you have trouble at dusk, see your doctor. And be very careful of sleeping pills, alcohol, tranquilizers, and other medications that may cause or worsen sundowning.

Chapter 5

Depression, Anxiety
& Unrest

It's been said, but bears repeating: The most common reason for sleeplessness is stress. The problem is not really how overpowering and dire the stress is, but how we react to it. Not all stress is negative, unless we let it become so. (See page 48 for a listing of events that most of us find stressful, to a degree.)

Life without stress is impossible, of course. Everyone has times of grief, disappointment, guilt, and anxiety. Such feelings are normal and we survive and get on with our lives.

When we let the feelings remain, when we can't seem to shake them, sleep suffers and it's time to take stock. In general, anxiety tends to be associated with difficulty in falling asleep and depression with difficulty in staying asleep. It's not quite that simple, but close to it.

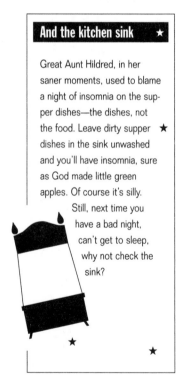

And the kitchen sink ★

Great Aunt Hildred, in her saner moments, used to blame a night of insomnia on the supper dishes—the dishes, not the food. Leave dirty supper ★ dishes in the sink unwashed and you'll have insomnia, sure as God made little green apples. Of course it's silly. Still, next time you have a bad night, can't get to sleep, why not check the sink?

And there's nothing wrong with feeling anxious or depressed. Anxiety and depression are nothing to ignore or be at all ashamed of. These days it seems unnecessary to point that out, but sleep specialists find that many people with insomnia don't even consider anxiety or depression as possibly contributing to lousy sleep, and seem reluctant to talk about it. Don't be reluctant. It's to your benefit to talk, because virtually all of these conditions can be treated and cured, or managed so you can get back on track.

Anxious About Anxiety?

Anxiety. How we let it rob us of sleep! Who hasn't gone to bed only to be kept awake by worries, stress responses, anxieties?

Those little worries can creep in and keep nudging us awake. The big worries seem easier to deal with. At least we know what they are and no one will blame us for being concerned about an operation coming up, about a key meeting next week to determine your job security, and the like. Who wouldn't be concerned?

Still, being concerned is one thing, being anxious and worried is another. People who seem to have their lives under reasonable control (and lose little sleep) are not free of stress or worries; they have found ways to handle their reactions. How? By utilizing some of the following techniques, available to all of us, and many covered elsewhere in this book:

• Be sure you get regular exercise and try for plenty of sunlight or, if necessary, bright light exposure.

• Stick to a good balanced diet.

• Stay with your good sleep hygiene—bedtime rituals, hot baths, proper snack, going to bed at about the same time each night, getting up at the same time each morning, and so on. Worry makes this difficult, but staying with it helps banish the worry.

• Think about how your worries started. Can't pin it down? Or was it a big event? Anxiety and depression sometimes are kicked off by a stressful event in the immediate past, or often a month or two earlier.

• Recognize that worries and anxiety are more likely to happen and disturb sleep in older people. But do not accept aging as a reason for the conditions. It's not, and treatment is indicated at any age.

• List your worries on paper, determine what you can do about them, and set the paper aside for the night. Sleeping will not solve your worries, but worry will upset your sleep if you let it.

• Talk to your spouse, your lover, your friend, your doctor—anyone you trust—and admit your fears and worries. Worry often is an outgrowth of fear, and some of us worry unnecessarily over irrational fears. It helps to get some feedback.

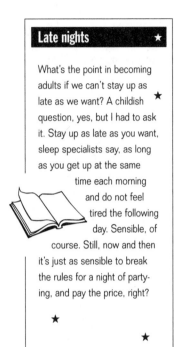

Late nights ★

What's the point in becoming adults if we can't stay up as late as we want? A childish ★ question, yes, but I had to ask it. Stay up as late as you want, sleep specialists say, as long as you get up at the same time each morning and do not feel tired the following day. Sensible, of course. Still, now and then it's just as sensible to break the rules for a night of partying, and pay the price, right?

★

★

Anxiety Attacks

Worry and anxiety overlap to a great extent, with one important difference. If you're worried, you need something to worry about. If you're filled with anxiety, you may or may not have an identifiable situation to be anxious about. Free-floating anxiety can be extremely upsetting.

You may be feeling fine, unburdened with overwhelming problems, when out of the blue you feel an overwhelming sense of terror, or acute anxiety. Much has been written about acute anxiety or panic attacks, but the root cause is still not completely understood.

I can testify to the immensity of such attacks—and to the great sense of relief after successful therapy, for they can be treated and cured or contained. For several years, I had such acute anxiety attacks, as often as two or three times a week.

Working in New York City and commuting from Connecticut, I found Grand Central Station a likely spot for these episodes, but they happened anywhere. The onset was sudden, with flushing, rapid heartbeat, rapid shallow breathing, hollow feeling of being about to soil my drawers (didn't happen), overwhelming feeling of sinking (especially on tile or concrete floors), of losing control, of being on another plane and not able to contact the people around me, even when walking with friends. Overshadowing all this was the knowledge that I was dying. That I did not die after repeated attacks had little effect; the next time the fear of death was just as strong.

If you have experienced a panic attack, you may recognize some or all of the symptoms (and there were more); if you haven't, good. These episodes left me hanging on the ropes, getting wildly fragmented sleep, and so on. But I found a way out. It took some looking and some doing. Over a couple of years I went through a series of counselors, with moderate to no help until finding a psychiatrist who came up with what I needed—regular low doses of imipramine (Tofranil) and good productive talks, along with an open invitation to call whenever I had questions.

This opened a new life, without question. I had become nearly housebound, not seeing friends, giving up social situations I enjoyed, spending nearly all of my time fearing the next attack. Within a month I was past that, and within 2 months, I was well on the way to normal living (including all its stresses and anxieties).

That was 15 to 20 years ago. I still take a low maintenance dose of imipramine daily. I talk about this because I know the pain and the frustration of free-floating anxiety. I also know it can be contained. And I'm happy to be able to relate this with no guilt, no hesitation. Statistically, panic attacks usually appear in your mid-20s, more often in women than in men. Mine appeared far later than that, and I'm male.

So, if you suspect your anxieties are getting out of hand, do not hesitate. See your doctor or counselor. Many people do not require medication, and respond to behavioral techniques such as relaxation, exercise, and cognitive therapy.

Edison's legacy ★

★
Yes, some famous people have slept little at night, getting by with short sleep and a few naps. Few gloated about it as Thomas Edison did, however, not exactly endearing himself to generations of insomniacs to come. He slept 3 or 4 hours a night, and was proud of it. Edison had no interest in 8 hours of sleep a night, calling it a ★ waste of time—"a heritage from our cave days." He wanted his electric lights to cut our dependency on a full night's sleep, and succeeded only too well. He has a lot to answer for.

★

Developed in 1965 by Dr. Thomas Holmes, a psychiatrist at the University of Washington, this list of stress producing events has been used by countless health care providers. Note that not all the events are negative, per se, yet all may lead to insomnia.

Stress Producing Events (in order of most to least stressfull)

- Death of a spouse
- Divorce
- Marital separation
- Jail term
- Death of a close family member
- Personal injury or illness
- Marriage
- Fired at work
- Reconciled with mate
- Retirement
- Changed health in family member
- Pregnancy
- Sex difficulties
- New family member
- Business readjustment
- Changed financial status
- Death of a close friend
- Changed to a different line of work
- Increased arguments with mate
- New mortgage or loan

- Foreclosure of mortgage or loan
- Changed work responsibility
- Child left home
- Trouble with in-laws
- Outstanding personal achievement
- Mate began or ended work
- Changed living conditions
- Revision of personal habits
- Trouble with boss
- Changed work hours or conditions
- Changed residence
- Changed schools
- Changed church activities
- Changed social activities
- Changed number of family meetings
- Changed eating habits
- Vacation
- Christmas
- Minor violation of law

Depression and Sleep

There's nothing unusual about feeling blue, feeling down, or grieving on occasion: the death of a loved one, death of your dog who's been loyally with you for 12 years, loss of understanding with an old friend.

Grief is natural. Prolonging it may not be. Watch for distorted thinking over sad events, as an indication of possible depression. And others may recognize this even if you do not. For example, if your spouse dies at age 60, no one would deny you your grief, which can last some time.

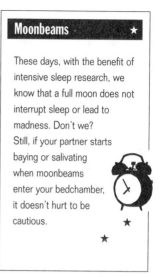

Moonbeams ★

These days, with the benefit of intensive sleep research, we know that a full moon does not interrupt sleep or lead to madness. Don't we?
Still, if your partner starts baying or salivating when moonbeams enter your bedchamber, it doesn't hurt to be cautious.

★
★

But if you think and say only "It's unfair, it's unfair; what will become of me?" rather than something like, "I miss him, I miss our living together," you may be looking at the event through some distortion. Sometimes depression follows changes in your life, such as loss of a job, retirement, death of a loved one (it used to be called situational depression), but more often, no single stressful happening started it. Remember that people have similar or identical events to deal with and not everyone develops depression.

Signs of Possible Depression:

• Early morning awakenings

• Loss of interest in friends and family

• Inability to make decisions

• Irrational disappointment in yourself as a person, as a partner, as a parent, as a worker

• Reluctance to look ahead and plan anything

• Poor appetite (or occasional binge eating)

- Loss of interest in sex

- Insomnia (occasionally oversleeping)

- Your sleep is often short and dream-filled (people with depression may drop quickly into REM sleep, and spend less than normal time in deep delta sleep)

If you identify with several of these points, you may have depression. What to do?

Admit it, and try to take steps to break the feelings. Try getting outside, into the country if you can. Buy yourself a loud, brightly colored shirt or scarf. Meet a friend for a picnic. Watch comedies on your VCR. Get closer to your pet. If you don't have a pet, how about getting one? Keep up on your diet. Get close to your family.

Above all, get adequate exercise, preferably outdoors, preferably vigorous aerobics that bring your endorphins into play—the body's feel-good substance. (See Chapter 9: Exercise and Relaxation.) You don't need to overwork, but doing something aerobic for 30 to 60 minutes three times a week—more if you want to—will help considerably.

Even if you don't feel like doing any of this—and you very well may not—do it anyway. Just go through the motions and take it on faith that they may help. With many depressive states that keep you from sleeping well at night or feeling well during the day, this is all you will need.

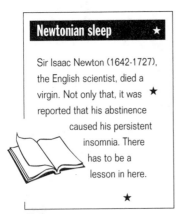

Newtonian sleep ★

Sir Isaac Newton (1642-1727), the English scientist, died a virgin. Not only that, it was ★ reported that his abstinence caused his persistent insomnia. There has to be a lesson in here.

★

If you feel or see no improvement over 2 or 3 weeks, or if your negative thoughts seem to be increasing, by all means, see your doctor. While some people have a slight predisposition for depression, the condition can be cured or contained in virtually everyone. Nearly all depression can be successfully treated—and should be.

Don't let it go unchecked—in you or in a loved one.

Chapter 6

Body Clocks Out of Sync

Sunday Night Insomnia

During the week, you get to bed at a reasonable time and get up every morning at 7. Then comes the weekend. Friday night you socialize and get to bed at 1 am, rather than your usual 11 pm. You sleep until 9 Saturday morning. You get 8 hours of sleep, but your body rhythm loses 2 hours. Your internal clock is 2 hours behind the clock on the wall. Saturday night you get to bed at midnight and you sleep until 8 Sunday morning. Another hour's loss for your body clock. You may feel tired and take a nap Sunday afternoon.

Sunday evening, you take yourself to task. Got to get to bed at 11; Monday's a workday.

You can't will yourself to sleep, although you try. It may be 11 pm by the clock on the wall, but your body clock thinks it is closer to 8, or a bit earlier depending on the nap. By the time your body clock catches up with your usual 11 pm bedtime, the clock on the wall says it's 2 am or later. You'll know, because you've probably been awake for those 3-plus hours.

Sunday night insomnia. The only reason it has a name is because it is so common. Sunday night problems are not necessarily because you hate the idea of going to work, although that may play a part. More likely, your sleep disruption plays a major part. How to avoid it? Go to bed later on weekends if you wish, but get up at your regular time. You may feel tired, but avoid the naps. Try to keep your body clock on its regular timing. It doesn't take weekends off.

Yes, it's tempting to stay up late and sleep in late on weekends (and other days), but giving in can result in major disruptions in your sleep-wake schedule. Most people, especially those with

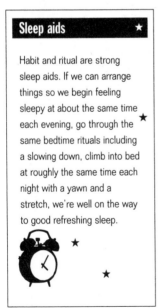

Sleep aids ★

Habit and ritual are strong sleep aids. If we can arrange things so we begin feeling sleepy at about the same time each evening, go through the ★ same bedtime rituals including a slowing down, climb into bed at roughly the same time each night with a yawn and a stretch, we're well on the way to good refreshing sleep.

regular daytime job schedules, cannot let this happen.

Circadian Clockworks

We have a constant adjustment going on between our body clocks and the clocks on the wall. Most of us, totally free of outside influences such as sunlight and darkness, tend to go to sleep at 25 hour intervals. (Sleep researchers have determined this, sometimes by checking fellow researchers living in a cave, voluntarily.)

Notice that we naturally fall asleep every 25 hours, not every 24. There are some fractions involved, but these basic numbers are true for most of us: We have to make up 1 hour each day, to stay synchronized with our 24-hour schedule that's not only accepted by society, but is caused by the rotation of the earth. Our morning get-out-of-bed time is probably the most important time signal our body clock uses to keep it all set correctly.

Slugabeds ★

From Home and Health (1879): An outstanding farmer said, "I do not care to have my men get up before five or half-past five in the morning. If they go to bed early and sleep soundly, they will do more work than if they got up at four or half-past four. We do not believe in the eight-hour law, but nevertheless are inclined to think that, as a general rule, we work too many hours on the farm." ★

This circadian rhythm within us is tied in with many body functions. It is responsible for organizing body processes so everything is in the right order. A simplified example: circadian rhythm will lower body temperature so a hormone will be released for a special task. That done, the rhythm will return the temperature, so other body functions can operate at their peak.

Our circadian clock is at work when we experience regular changes of body temperature dipping in the very early morning hours and rising to the late forenoon. The range is no more than some 2 degrees F, and appreciably less in most older people, but the effect, sleep specialists are discovering, can be remarkable.

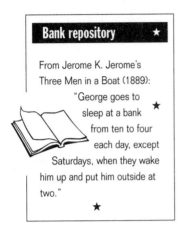

Bank repository ★

From Jerome K. Jerome's
Three Men in a Boat (1889):
"George goes to
sleep at a bank ★
from ten to four
each day, except
Saturdays, when they wake
him up and put him outside at
two."

★

Regulation by our body clocks can affect sleep, hunger, alertness, our mood, our sexual drive, nearly every body function to some degree. When our body clock malfunctions, it often results in a disruption of our sleep-wake schedule.

If you take nights of good sleep for granted, you're one of the lucky ones. With circadian rhythm to contend with, plus the balance between REM and non-REM sleep, plus the wide variety of medical, emotional, and physical surrounding influences, the wonder is not that we occasionally have poor sleep, but that we often have good sleep.

Night Owls and Larks

People's circadian rhythms do differ. Some few people, for example, don't get sleepy until 3 or 4 am and will sleep comfortably until noon. Delayed sleep phase syndrome, it's called. These are the extreme night owls.

Such people—and some writers are in this camp—will work well from about 6 in the evening to 2 in the morning, then sleep until noon, or close to it. This is fine, if you can do your work this way and are not tied to a 9-to-5 workday, and do not mind being out of sync with society— working while most people sleep, sleeping while most people (including your family?) are up and about.

Larks, on the other hand—morning people—tend to go to bed early and get up early, eager, ready to go (and a real challenge for those of us whose rhythms tend to have us crawling out at a reasonable hour rather than vaulting out of bed before the crack of dawn . . . but I editorialize).

Keep in mind that while some people are strongly morning or night people, probably genetically determined, most of us do not have such strong leanings either way. That doesn't mean we are immune to sleep-wake disturbances, not at all.

We can bring them on by putting ourselves through wild time changes and schedule alterations. We may go to bed at 10 one evening, 3 am the next night, midnight the next night, and so on. Once in awhile this has to be done, but be this lax about bedtime for a couple of weeks or months, and you'll have trouble getting to sleep no matter what time you go to bed, with your body not knowing what the schedule is. And this is without even leaving home. We also do it with the jet lag of travel, the effects of working irregular shifts, and more.

Our circadian rhythms often change with age. Middle-aged and older people tend to have shorter body clock schedules, which makes them morning people. Older people may be ready for bed at, say, 8 or 9 in the evening, and if they heed the call and turn in, they may awaken at 3 or 4 in the morning, or earlier. (See Chapter 4: Sleep Changes with Aging.) A short body clock schedule can happen at any age, of course. Most people do not want this sort of a sleep-wake schedule that leaves them out of touch with others, or at least on different schedules. The patterns may be adjusted through light therapy or chronotherapy (see below).

Clock Therapy

What to do about an off-center sleep pattern? Chronotherapy has been used for some years in helping us reset our body clocks, and is usually effective, although it may seem a bit drastic. If you think it will help with your delayed sleep pattern, say, try the treatment during vacation or sick leave and with supervision. Most of us would like our doctor's approval—or that of a sleep specialist—before beginning. It takes resolve and you'll have your internal clock changing for perhaps a week.

In essence, if you have been sleeping from 4 am to noon, you will go to bed 3 hours later on the first day of therapy. Yes, later. Chronotherapy is based on the next day, not the previous day. So, you will go to sleep at 7 am and set your alarm for 3 pm. The next day you go to sleep at 10 am and set your alarm for 6 pm. You keep advancing your bedtime by 3 hours each day, always setting the alarm for 8 hours hence. And no napping.

A recipe for internal clock mixup? Exactly, and that's part of the therapy. You need to get unstuck before you can have your body clock reset. You keep doing these daily adjustments until you are close to what you want as a regular sleep schedule. On the sixth day, for example, you should be going to bed at 10 pm and sleeping until 6 am. Make it 11 pm to 7 am if you wish, and stick with it.

Some people have a difficult time staying with the new schedule, while others find it comparatively easy. If you find it hard, you may have to do another session of chronotherapy for better results.

Light Therapy

This treatment of a fast or slow internal clock is based on the therapeutic advantages of light, and is well accepted. Sunlight is a major way our body's clock is set, so exposure to bright light has been found to shift the circardian phase. It can reverse the sleep-wake cycle of a shift worker, and realign a sleep-wake cycle that is not that far off the norm.

Light is now known to be so important that sleep specialists recommend getting into the sunlight, or at least outside, for at least a half hour a day, whatever your sleep problem. And if you have none, do it anyway as a preventive measure.

Outside light does the most good in the morning, and an ideal situation is to step onto the patio first thing after getting up, and bask in the sunlight. Most of us lack these ideal conditions, but it does help to be out even if it's later in the day and cloudy. Try to stay out for an hour in those circumstances and couple it with some exercise. (See Chapter 9: Exercise and Relaxation.)

The outdoor light can be replaced or augmented by bright lights indoors, which has proven helpful for many sufferers of altered sleep patterns as well as persons who have seasonal affective disorder (SAD). SAD includes prolonged sleep, depression, lethargy, and other symptoms.

To use bright light therapy and gain better sleep, you purchase or construct a light box with very high illumination—at least 2,500 lux, which is far more than ordinary room light (150 to 200 lux) but less than bright sunshine (100,000 lux). Don't bother turning on all your regular room lights; they will not do the job.

To take the light box treatment, preferably in the morning, sit 3 feet from the light box for 15 to 30 minutes. Vary your exposure with how you feel. If you feel too wired, cut down your exposure. If you feel little effect, increase it.

Sleep specialists differ in their recommended exposure times, from 15 minutes to an hour or two. This is another treatment that you do at home, but check with your doctor to be sure you're on the best program, with the right kind of light box and the right length of exposure. Once you get it right, you'll keep on with it as a daily part of your routine, so take some time in the beginning. Some people have constructed their own light boxes from four shop lights each containing two 4-foot fluorescent tubes and hanging the unit from their ceiling. Here again, I wouldn't make my own, but you may be comfortable doing such things.

For information about light therapy, including names of practitioners and information on light boxes, contact The Society for Light Treatment and Biological Rhythms, 10200 W 44th Ave, Suite 304, Wheat Ridge, CO 80033. The SLTBR is a nonprofit professional association.

Instant naps

In the old days, Dad came ★ home from the gas station for noon dinner. That finished, he stretched out on the living room davenport, fell immediately asleep, awoke in 15 minutes, and went back to work refreshed. As a youngster, I marveled at this routine, but a recent conversation with a friend shakes my admiration a bit. When he was a boy on the farm, his dad came in from the fields for noontime dinner (the big meal always at midday, when it was needed), then stayed in the kitchen chair sitting bolt upright and slept for 15 minutes. My friend spent many a noontime in the summers waiting for the old man to fall, but he never did. He awoke refreshed and went back to the fields. ★

★

Jet Lag

Jet lag, a modern phenomenon, is a good example of a sleep-wake disturbance in miniature—a classic case with known causes and some proven remedies.

The mechanism is well-known by now, with air travel so common. And the main problem is excessive daytime sleepiness. If you don't mind being in a fog for a few days after traveling across time lines and have no tight schedule to keep, you may not mind jet lag. Most of us do.

The routine: Say you live in California and fly to New York, which is 3 hours ahead of California time. If you have dinner at your usual time, say 6, your body still is on California time and feels that it's 3 in the afternoon, not the right time for dinner. If you go to bed at your usual time of 11, your body feels that it's 8 and you're likely to lie there staring at the ceiling.

All of us know the drill. And it can be much worse if you fly over several time changes, to Europe, for example. By the way, traveling from east to west presents far less of an adaptation problem because we're gaining hours, not losing them.

If you must travel from Chicago to London, for example, your problem depends somewhat on why you're going. It takes most people 2 or 3 days to readjust on landing, and most of us are not at our most acute during the readjustment phase. Scientists have studied this on travelers, including horses. All took time to regain their peak alertness and performance, even the horses. (Racehorses, that is, which sound like the jet-lagged ones I wagered on in my younger days.)

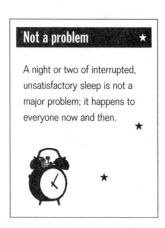

Not a problem ★

A night or two of interrupted, unsatisfactory sleep is not a major problem; it happens to everyone now and then. ★

So if your mission is vital, try to arrive a day or two early, before the meeting, the concert where you're performing, the race you're going to win at the Derby. If this is impractical, try these recommendations:

On the day you fly, say from New York to London, board the plane, drink no alcohol, drink plenty of water, and sleep all you can. This may take a firm hand with attendants, so they will indeed not wake you up for free drinks, snacks, extra blankets, and so on.

Do wake up and have a good breakfast at 7 am London time, then stay awake and walk around on the plane while you can. On arrival, follow the meal pattern in London, get to bed a little early but not as soon as you've landed. This routine, once you know it, is not as cumbersome as it sounds and should have you better adjusted by the second day.

Drinking lots of water is important, to counter dehydration from the dry conditions in the plane. Dehydration may hinder the adjustments of your body rhythms.

Light and darkness contribute to jet lag too. If you leave New York on a bright afternoon and arrive in London in the early hours of a dark and rainy morning, your body's going to wonder What now? But proper eating, getting aboard the local times, and trying for some bright lights all help.

A basic approach to preventing or mitigating jet lag is simply to try to adjust to the mealtimes and sleep times of the country you're heading for, a few days before you leave. If the whole plan is not possible, any of the steps you can take will help.

Shiftwork

More than 22 million Americans now work something other than a traditional day shift, and the total seems to be increasing. Full-time night shift work is difficult and demands adjustment since our bodies are programmed for sleep then. Even more problems, it seems, come to those who rotate shifts.

Changing shift workers (police officers, hospital staff, airline workers, nurses, media personnel, and many others) may rotate every few weeks from day shift (11 am to 7 pm), to evening shift (7 pm to 3 am), then night shift (3 am to 11 am). The changes at least are forward rather than backward, somewhat easing our ability to cope, but it does take a week or two for most of us to adjust to a new shift.

It's no wonder that, in general, shift or night workers have a higher than average incidence of sleep problems, injuries, accidents, stress-related problems with the cardiovascular and gastrointestinal systems.

And the concern over accidents and poor judgment calls during sleep-deprived hours is growing. The National Sleep Foundation and the Association of Professional Sleep Societies have studied the problem and issued warnings: most people have trouble functioning at their best during early morning hours (2 to 7 am) and in the afternoon (2 to 5 pm) although less pronouncedly. Further, if we're deprived of sleep, the decrease in abilities to function at those approximate times is greater, and undoubtedly contributes to some of the accident figures.

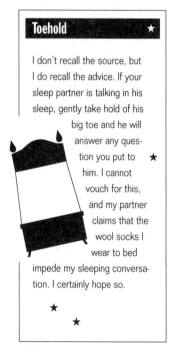

Toehold ★

I don't recall the source, but I do recall the advice. If your sleep partner is talking in his sleep, gently take hold of his big toe and he will answer any question you put to ★ him. I cannot vouch for this, and my partner claims that the wool socks I wear to bed impede my sleeping conversation. I certainly hope so.

★

★

This is a justifiable concern, and various groups are trying to cut back on some of the sleep loss—cutting down the maximum hours on duty of medical residents, airline pilots, and others. Examples of serious accidents that seem to be time-related are well-known by now—the Chernobyl and Three Mile Island nuclear power plant incidents, the Exxon Valdez grounding, the clustering of car accidents around the early morning poor functioning times, and the like.

If you are on a shift schedule, what can you do to remain on top of things? First, insist on your sleep times during the day and make sure your family and friends know it's sacrosanct. A visit from your friendly insurance salesman at noon is like a visit to a day worker at 3 am.

Driving home from shift work, wear dark glasses so the light will not further wake you. Be sure you take time to wind down and make it a habit to go through the usual bedtime routines. (See Chapter 7: How's Your Sleep Hygiene?) Make sure your bedroom is darkened and as soundproof as you can make it. Use white noise machines, soft ear plugs, eye masks—anything that will help you sleep soundly.

Try to maintain this regular sleep schedule 7 days a week, even when there are times you'd rather toss your schedule over for time with your family or friends on the weekend.

Unfortunately, there are no magic answers to the night shift challenges because the human body is in basic rebellion. Some people find it easier than others, younger people generally find it easier than others. If you have sleep problems that you can't solve, get in touch with your doctor and talk about it. See the list of approved sleep clinics (on page 131) for professional help near you.

Chapter 7

How's Your Sleep Hygiene?

Sleep specialists had to come up with their own jargon because no one had done this work before. But sleep hygiene? My well-thumbed desk dictionary defines hygiene as "A science of the establishment and maintenance of health" or "Conditions or practices (as of cleanliness) conducive to health."

So yes, it does make sense. Sleep hygiene covers a range of things to do and not do that will give you a better than average shot at healthful sleep—and the energy that comes with it. Here's where you really take charge. Give good sleep a top priority; no one can do it for you. The recommendations are clear and based on common sense as well as on scientific findings.

Cut Out the Big Three

Reduce caffeine, limit alcohol, and get rid of nicotine. There's just no denying it, if you partake of coffee, tea, chocolate, cola, booze, and if you smoke, you will sleep much better without those delights (and improve your general health). Sounds like a bitter price to pay? Think about those sleepless nights and dragged-out days that brought you to this book in the first place.

Most sleep specialists know that total abolition may be impossible for some of us, and not always necessary, but you'll have trouble convincing anyone that you can go merrily along with old bad habits and achieve decent sleep. If you smoke, you know that the nicotine in tobacco is a stimulant, as is caffeine in coffee, cola, and tea. Studies leave no doubt: people who smoke (or chew tobacco) are likely to have both kinds of insomnia—trouble getting to sleep and trouble staying asleep.

They have trouble getting to sleep because the nicotine raises blood pressure, increases the heart rate and stimulates brain wave activity—three conditions that don't invite good sleep. Smokers in general have more fragmented sleep than nonsmokers, which also may mean they get less of the deep restorative sleep. Nicotine withdrawal symptoms and drying out of nasal mucosa lead to smokers waking up more often, once asleep.

No one claims that giving up smoking is always easy, but we can't really make a case for smoking, poor sleep or no. Millions of Americans have stopped. Do it. And note that you'll get sleep benefits even as you still have daytime cigarette-withdrawal symptoms, if they occur.

Mark Twain, who said most of the things worth remembering in this country's history, smoked cheap, powerful cigars, but didn't let it become a habit. "I can stop anytime I want to," he said. "In fact, I've done it a thousand times." Twain, a lifelong insomniac, also admitted in his later years that he had to watch what he ate or his sleep would be violated. "I've had to give up toying with mince pie after midnight," he said. Twain is hardly a role model for temperate living, but he does provide a perspective that sometimes helps, continually fresh and sardonic.

Wet towel ★

From Home and Health (1879): To cure sleeplessness, "Wet half a towel, apply it to the back of the neck, pressing it upward toward the base of the brain, and fasten the dry half of the towel over so as to ★ prevent too-rapid exhalation." It is suggested that this method is a special boon to those who suffer from over-excitement of the brain. And presumably not much of a boon to your bed partner. ★ ★

If you drink coffee or tea or soda, practice moderation. Some of us dismiss the effects of caffeine, but it is a powerful stimulant. Think of how well it works as a pickup to overcome fatigue. Some people find it nearly impossible to get started in the morning without a cup or two of caffeine-laden coffee. No decaf for these addicts. But the desired effect in the morning works in reverse when you try to sleep after too much caffeine. Remember, caffeine is present not only in coffee but also in tea, in chocolate, and in many medications including some nonprescription drugs. The following chart shows a few examples of how easy it is to pile up caffeine from different sources. Remember, too, that there are worthy alternatives. Decaf coffee is much more flavorful than it used to be, herbal teas without caffeine are fine any time, especially if you want something in the evening, and some sodas are available without caffeine; check the labels.

How much is too much? If you take on 250 to 300 milligrams and more during the day, you may be on your way to caffeine addiction, and you're certainly courting rocky nights. And that's just three or four cups of regular coffee during the entire day.

Sample Caffeine Content of Drinks, Foods, Drugs

Coffee (5-ounce cup)

Drip method	115 mg
Percolator	80
Instant	65
Decaf	2-3

Tea (5-ounce cup)

Steeped	40 mg
Instant	30
Iced tea (10 ounce glass)	70

Chocolate

Cocoa (5-ounce cup)	4 mg
Chocolate bar (6 ounces)	25

Soft drinks

Coca-cola	46 mg
Diet Coke	46
Pepsi-Cola	38
Diet Pepsi	36
Dr. Pepper	40
RC Cola	36
Mountain Dew	54

Nonprescription Drugs, Caffeine Content

No Doz (alertness)	100 mg
Vivarin (alertness)	200
Dexatrim (weight control)	200
Excedrin (pain relief)	65
Anacin (pain relief)	2
Triaminicin tablets (cold/allergy)	30
Dristan tablets (cold/allergy)	16

It's true that reaction to stimulants varies widely among individuals. A cup of regular coffee will send one person into orbit and have little apparent effect on another. Older persons are apt to be affected more by stimulants, as well as by other medications. But 250 to 300 mg of caffeine a day is the limit for most of us. Too much caffeine and we get shaky, on edge, irritable, have heart palpitations, nausea, diarrhea, frequent urination, other symptoms . . . leading to insomnia (which is a symptom in itself, of course).

If you drink alcohol, use caution and do not take it as a sleeping aid. It's that simple. Yes, doctors used to prescribe a nightcap—a whiskey and hot water, a glass of port—but it really does not help you sleep well. We don't all react the same, of course. Some people find a drink before bedtime does help them fall asleep; others find it makes falling asleep more difficult. But both groups end up with fragmented sleep and frequent awakenings.

It's not necessary to become a teetotaler. If you enjoy a glass of wine or two with your evening meal, fine. But if you're in the habit of having more drinks during the evening, or even a drink or two just

Plants help ★

Place elderberries under your pillow for a better chance of good sound sleep, but I suppose you knew that. How about this one: Lay mistletoe near your bedroom door and kiss your sleep worries goodbye! Too delicate? Well, rub lettuce juice onto your forehead and prepare for record-breaking sleep. (As long as your sleep partner concurs.)

★   ★

before bedtime, cut them out. The dinnertime alcohol probably will be out of your bloodstream by bedtime, but the late drink will not. A drink within an hour or two of going to bed can cause the light fragmented sleep and awakenings that leave you drained.

In short, using booze to snooze is not a good idea. Sleep patterns in chronic alcoholics are abnormal—fragmented and shallow. And alcoholics actually get precious little deep restorative sleep or REM sleep.

Drinks at bedtime also can start or aggravate sleep apnea (see Chapter 12: Sleep Disorders, Parasomnias, et al.), by relaxing throat and upper airway musculature. So can some sleeping pills, so always let your doctor know if you have trouble with heavy snoring, one of the first signs. One controlled study shows that sleep apnea episodes were five times more likely in men when they consumed significant amounts of alcohol.

Some texts go into detail on ways to minimize or eliminate drinking as a sleep problem, but a practical test is easy: If you take a drink or two before retiring and have sleep problems, give up the drinks for a week and see for yourself how your sleep compares. Keep absolute track of your alcoholic drinks—wine, beer, cocktails, highballs—to see how much you do consume if you have any doubt. Obviously, total honesty is necessary here. Can you give up the late night drinks with no problem? Can you give up taking a drink or two to get back to sleep once you awaken at night? Any private doubts about your control?

If you need help, it's available through organizations like Alcoholics Anonymous, hospital programs, private counseling, and more. A lot of us can reassure you that it can be done, but the decision is up to you.

Boring naps ★

"A nap, my friend, is a brief period of sleep which overtakes superannuated persons when they endeavour to entertain unwelcome visitors or to listen to scientific lectures."
—George Bernard Shaw ★

★

Practical Sleep Hygiene Tips

Consider the bedtime rituals we come up with for young children. The relaxing bath, the warm fuzzy pajamas, the winding down time with a story (the same story for the 200th time?), the tucking into bed, the hugs. . . . No wonder kids sleep well after that preparation.

So now that we're big and adult, is there any reason to deny ourselves those warm fuzzy pleasures? Absolutely not. In fact, developing an evening ritual of your own, preparing yourself, is one of the most important ways to achieve more and better sleep. Here's a brief list of recommendations:

- DO go to bed each night at the same time. (An occasional night staying up late is no problem.) In the old days in Granite Falls, Minnesota (sorry you didn't all know Granite Falls) 75 percent of the citizenry listened to Cedric Adams's nightly news on WCCO radio, then retired at 10:15. It may have been 100 percent; we didn't poll people in those far-off times; we let them sleep.

- DO get up at the same time each morning. If you need to vary sleep time, adjust your bedtime, not wake up time.

- DO get regular exercise, but not within 4 hours of going to bed. Late afternoon is better, or early morning if necessary. (See Chapter 9: Relaxation & Exercise.)

- DO eat at regular times, and eat very little in the evening before bedtime. Overall diet is important for good sleep as well as all-around good health. Some sleep specialists advise having your heavy meal at noon rather than in the evening if you can, heeding "The later the meal, the lighter the meal." In the old days, most everyone did this, unaware that we were scientifically correct. (See Chapter 8: Eat Right, Sleep Tight.)

- DO set aside a few minutes each evening to jot down your immediate problems and what you plan to do about them, if you know. Talk over mutual concerns with your partner if you can. This worry time is designed to help you avoid carrying problems to bed. Simple as it sounds, it does seem to work. And keep a note pad and pencil on your nightstand to jot down those nagging thoughts or ideas that may keep you awake. Writers are notorious note scribblers, but don't look to writers as models of sane sleep.

- DO use your bedroom just for sleep—and sex, if it is a loving relationship. Years ago, bedrooms were called sleeping rooms—and no, I don't know if they were also called sex rooms, but I doubt it. Come on now. Sex certainly is a lovely way to get sleepy. But if one partner sees it as a duty, better not. At any age. A common misconception (pardon the word) about old age, is that those attaining it lose interest in sex. Wrong. We may prefer a different style, with less swinging from the chandelier and more stroking, but the older folks I know realize that we have delightful times . . . and no kids around.

- DO make sure your bedroom is conducive to sleep—a comfortable bed, quiet darkened room at a comfortable temperature. Most people sleep best in about 65 degrees. At about 75 and up, it gets too warm for comfortable sleep and lower than 60, we're less likely to sleep long enough to feel rested. We can fall asleep in well lighted areas, but far easier if the room is dark; bright light tells our bodies to wake up. And we can fall asleep on a board, but far easier on a comfortable mattress; this varies by person, as do the kinds of sheets, night clothes (if any), pillows, and blankets.

- DO take measures to solve obvious sleep problems. If your bedroom is noisy and lighter than you desire, hang some heavy draperies, use more rugs and carpet to soak up sound. Tell your neighbors to stop playing the bagpipes after midnight. Investigate a white noise machine, or soothing woodland-seashore tapes that help mask sound. Try an eyemask if you want it darker.

- DO ease your way into bed with a relaxing routine. A hot bath is right for some, with sleep easier as your body cools down. A glass of warm milk or herbal tea with crackers may work. Or a favorite book or soothing music. Trial and error will help you decide.

- DO NOT watch the clock. If you need to set an alarm clock, do so, but put it in a drawer or under your bed. Few things are more frustrating than awakening in the night and staring at the dial or digital face of a clock.

- DO NOT use your bedroom for sustained television viewing, paperwork from the office or home, paying bills, and the like.

- DO NOT eat a heavy meal in the evening, even when you dine out. It takes up to 5 hours to clear the stomach. One nearly sure-fire way to produce insomnia is to scarf down a super pizza with everything and a beer while watching the late show.

- DO NOT lie in bed waiting to fall asleep for more than, say, 30 minutes. Then get up, go to another room, read a light book, listen to music, have a cup of herbal tea—and try again later. Try not to associate the bedroom with frustration.

- DO NOT go to bed until you're sleepy. This may mean adjusting the time you go to bed.

- DO NOT lie awake, willing yourself to sleep. Can't be done. You need to relax and let it come. Try whatever works for you—thinking sublime thoughts, holding your teddy bear (no one but your partner need know), praying, feeling the peace of mind in knowing you're wearing your sleepiest pajamas. Sure, it can be a little crazy. The only crazier thing is not being able to fall asleep.

Breathe Right® strips ★

Few sleep aids gain national appeal through the activity of professional football players. The Breathe Right nasal strip has done just that, prompting high sales of this over-the-counter device and reports of better breathing and better sleep. Athletes use it to increase their airways for better breathing during the game; not better sleep.

The Breathe Right is two plastic strips, with adhesive on one side. It works mechanically. Apply one across the bridge of your nose as directed and as the plastic strips gradually straighten, they increase the flare of each nostril. Wear it at night, or any time you want easier nasal breathing. Medical studies of the device are underway, and until more information is available, the FDA has approved the company's claim that the strips "may reduce nasal airflow resistance."

- DO NOT become a slave to your sleep goals. If you go to bed at 10 pm and regularly lie awake until 11, it just makes sense to stay up an extra hour and go to bed at 11. Be sure you get up at your usual time.

- DO NOT get overly worried about some lost sleep. No one ever died from insomnia, but worrying about insomnia has kept many a person from decent sleep.

- DO NOT use alcohol as a bedtime sedative. (See above). Also, DO NOT take sleeping pills unless prescribed by your doctor. Get your doctor's advice on nonprescription pills too. (See Chapter 10: The Limited Role of Sleeping Pills.)

- DO NOT worry if your sleeping partner sleeps soundly through a noise that jars you wide awake. No two people have the same tolerance for noise, light, or other stimuli.

- DO NOT let the cat or dog sleep in your bedroom, unless you cannot stand to be parted for 8 hours. They're seldom any help and often a hindrance.

Mindgames ★

Several friends report that mental games do work when their body is tired but mind is racing. Two suggestions: ★

★

Yes, count sheep—or turtles, or birds, or zebras and distract both halves of your brain by picturing what they look like as you count them.

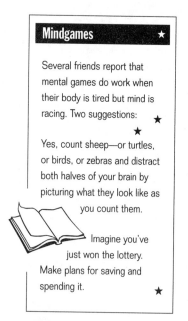

Imagine you've just won the lottery. Make plans for saving and spending it. ★

Bedtime—Choosing a Bed

Time to check your bed? It probably is, if you've had it for 10 years and more, or if it no longer feels comfortable. Keep in mind that you will spend one-third of your life in bed, sleeping or trying to get to sleep, so the bed deserves a close look. Check the following:

- One bed or two? If you sleep with a partner, this is a prime question. Sleeping in one bed brings its share of elbows in the ribs, kicks, turnings, nighttime commotion. Studies show that most people will get more deep sleep in a single bed than with a partner in a double. But most couples like the intimacy and the comfortable feeling of having thier partner close. We willingly give up some privacy in return for the warm feeling of togetherness. The choice is yours. And his or hers.

- Buy a bigger bed? Even if you're both good sleepers, you still move at least a dozen times a night. If you have trouble with sleep, the back-and-forth movement may be more than you want. One solution is a bigger bed. When a couple sleeps on a regular double bed, each has about the same space width as a baby's crib. Most couples opt for queen or king-size beds. (A twin bed is 39 by 75 or 80 inches, a double bed is 54 by 75 or 80 inches, a queen bed is 60 by 80 inches, a king bed is 76 by 80 inches, and a California king-size is 72 by 84 inches.)

- One solution to privacy versus intimacy is using two twin beds side by side, or two half-size mattresses on one large box spring, reducing the shock waves when your partner turns over.

- Is your mattress lumpy? Does it sag at the edges? Has it lost its resiliency, leaving you feeling lost in a cocoon? Time to look for a new one.

- What kind of new one? You'll find a wide variety when you begin looking at mattresses. Most people prefer an innerspring mattress, some like a foam mattress, some like a waterbed. Air-supported mattresses are now available.

- If you want an innerspring mattress, check out the firmness, not by listening to a salesperson, but by lying down on the mattress in the store, bouncing, testing. Do it with your partner, if it's to be shared. The tighter the coils and thicker the wire, the firmer the support. Don't get an innerspring with rock-like firmness unless you really want that feeling; we seem to have a penchant for FIRM mattresses, which can leave us with contact mainly at the pressure points (hips, shoulders) and too often these parts alone go to sleep. Look for a feeling of buoyancy, a cradling sensation, an even pressure over your whole body. The right mattress should support you in roughly the same position as when you are standing with good posture.

- If you want foam, the heavier the firmer. Foam mattresses can be used on a box spring or a specially designed platform. Some people with back problems prefer foam mattresses.

- If you want a waterbed, get the waveless kind with baffles and a heating element. Without the baffles, some people experience too many waves and nausea. Some pregnant women find waterbeds comfortable.

- One new bed idea you may want to check into is an air support style, available with two separate controls for firmness. Be prepared to pay more than you would think of for a bed. That holds true for innersprings too, that range from moderate to fancy pricing.

- When picking an innerspring, look for one at least 7 inches thick, with a minimum of 300 coils for full size, 375 for queen, and 450 for king, says the Better Sleep Council. While you want comfort, if your lower back, hips and shoulders sink into the mattress, that in itself can lead to morning backache.

- Some people, especially those with myalgia or backache, report convoluted mattress pads as helpful. These are hypoallergenic foam pads with a waffle-like texture, and are reasonably priced so you can give them a try.

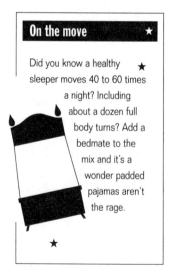

On the move ★

Did you know a healthy ★ sleeper moves 40 to 60 times a night? Including about a dozen full body turns? Add a bedmate to the mix and it's a wonder padded pajamas aren't the rage.

★

- Pillow talk. The kind is up to you: foam, feather, goose down. If you are allergic to some materials, this of course will guide your choice of pillow, and of the mattress. Don't get pillows that are too thick, just because they pile up nicely when you want to read. They may be too thick for good sleeping. And try the contour pillows if you wish, available in a variety of shapes, designed to hold your neck and head in good positions.

- And bedding? Your choice. Most people find cotton, and especially percale cotton sheets comfortable, and cotton blankets preferred to synthetic or wool. You like a bright red wool blanket? Use it. But know that most people prefer cotton and prefer neutral colors as better sleep promoters.

A good bed is important, but keep it all in perspective. People in other cultures sleep on the floor or on wooden frames or in hammocks. Do what you can to give yourself a bed that promotes sleep, but try not to make bed selection another problem you lose sleep over.

Chapter 8

Eat Right, Sleep Tight

One key to good sleep is a healthful diet. And the key to a healthful diet is moderation.

Our forefathers—some of them—knew this, long before the medical and nutrition folks began issuing almost weekly reports on the latest findings: Eat more oats. Don't eat more oats. Abolish eggs from your diet. Eat more eggs. Lettuce causes cancer. Lettuce is good for you. Eat fiber.

And so on. At times, it's hard to think of anything that has been cleared by all interested parties. Still, my grandparents ate well, and Grandma supplied not only all the cooking, but also the advice on nutrition, from experience. Some foods didn't sit well, and she knew it.

All foods coming out of her kitchen were started from scratch. She had bins of flour, bins of sugar, bins of potatoes and onions. No prepared food, no cake mixes, frozen foods, concentrates, additives. It was a glorious time for her grandsons, and I was one.

We had no problems with dining out at restaurants; we just didn't do it, whereas today, the average American eats at least four meals a week in restaurants, many in fast food establishments where, it's safe to say, the emphasis is on fried and flavorful. There were a few rules at Grandma's: Eat enough but don't stuff, drink water with the meals, take time for a good breakfast, and don't take more than you're going to eat (this was tough). It worked. We ate well and slept well.

Today, good nutrition is trickier, but no less important. Good sleep hinges on your overall good condition, so basic diet is important. We see this connection in reverse at times. That is, some people on a weight-loss diet that does not contain enough nutrients do indeed have sleep problems— insomnia, depression, fatigue, and the like.

The Pyramid Approach

The common American diet—what most of us really eat—is not the best way to combat or prevent insomnia. Typically, we eat far too much sugar (sugared cereal, pie, sweet rolls), too much fat (gravies, rich meat, puddings), and too few fresh vegetables, fruits, whole grain breads. You've heard it before? It still seems to be true. What Americans really eat is causing heart attacks, cancer, and insomnia—insomnia from being overweight, having high blood pressure, and overtaxing our digestive systems at night, trying to catch up with those large and heavy meals. Instead of concentrating on steak, French fries, milk shakes, and cheese cake, the closer we can come to a diet of fruit, vegetables, whole grain breads and cereals, legumes, fish, poultry, and occasional lean meat, the better we'll be.

Instead of demanding deep fried, skillet fried, any kind of fried foods, we will be so much better off when we think first of raw foods—raw vegetables or fruit—and then roasted, baked, steamed, boiled, broiled, or poached foods. Forget fried.

You must be familiar with the food guide pyramid (see page 80), charting an approach to better nutrition. It has the blessing of the U.S. Department of Agriculture, the Surgeon General, the American Heart Association, and the American Cancer Society, for starters. So, following these guidelines just makes good sense. Also, it's something you can safely try by yourself. And it's not the end of joyful eating.

> ### No pain, no gain ★
>
> Don't be surprised if you are sore for a few days after ★ changing from a soft mattress to a very firm one. It takes 3 to 5 days for your body to adjust to a new mattress, but in the long run your spine will be better supported when you sleep.
>
> ★

These are guidelines, remember. You're not going to keel over if you have five servings instead of the minimum recommendation of six from the bread, cereal, rice, and pasta group. Nor will a few extra servings of fruit or cheese set you up for trouble.

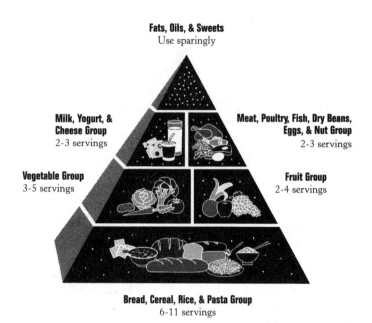

Fats, Oils, & Sweets
Use sparingly

**Milk, Yogurt, &
Cheese Group**
2-3 servings

**Meat, Poultry, Fish, Dry Beans,
Eggs, & Nut Group**
2-3 servings

Vegetable Group
3-5 servings

Fruit Group
2-4 servings

Bread, Cereal, Rice, & Pasta Group
6-11 servings

If you habitually have 10 servings from the fats and oil group and next to nothing from the fruit and vegetable groups, you're courting trouble—and sleepless nights. A few recommendations:

- With sleep a consideration, try to eat a basic breakfast, a substantial lunch, and a light evening dinner containing protein such as fish or poultry. Avoid heavy, spicy, rich meals at day's end. Aim for "the later, the lighter" meals.

- Eat a lot of fresh vegetables and fruit. With the large variety available throughout the year, we really have little excuse for avoiding them. So the cost is a consideration? When figuring what it will cost, remember to deduct what you pay for prepackaged, salted, low-nutrition munchies. So much of our eating is governed by habit. For a couple of weeks, be sure to have fresh fruit around—pears, apples, oranges, grapefruit, grapes, and on and on. Reach for fruit instead of a munchy; it's not the end of the world.

- When you eat the bulk of your food—from the bread, cereal, rice and pasta group—make it whole grain breads, unsweetened cereals, brown or whole rice. Not only are these better for you than white rice, sweet cereal, white bread, but also, they taste good. The taste, as well as the nutrients, haven't been processed out.

- Avoid too much fat. It's not that difficult, and the effects are worth it. Trim the fat off meat before cooking it, cut back on your red meat consumption (once or twice a week is fine, and no great sacrifice), get used to 2% or skim milk (I confess to gagging on skim, but finding 2% acceptable). And, cut back on ice cream, candies, cookies not just for the sugar saving, but also for the fat. It's hiding in a lot of sweets.

Don't be thrown by the number of "servings" recommended. My first reaction to lists like the food guide pyramid is to shrug and say to myself that I cannot possibly eat that many total servings . . . of anything. Not in one day. Not in one lifetime.

But study that list. A serving is generally a lot less than what we see on our plates. A serving of rice, for example, is 1/2 cup cooked (not much). A serving of bread is one slice, so any kind of a sandwich automatically gives you two of the six servings recommended from the bread group. Toast in the morning brings it to four. The servings add up in a hurry because they're smaller than you may think.

What Counts as a Serving?

Bread, cereal, rice, and pasta group

—1 slice of bread

—1 ounce of ready-to-eat cereal (1 ounce=1/4 cup to 2 cups depending on cereal)

—1/2 cup cooked cereal, rice, or pasta

—1/2 hamburger roll, bagel, or English muffin

—3 or 4 plain crackers (small)

Vegetable group

—1 cup of raw, leafy vegetables

—1/2 cup of other vegetables, cooked or chopped raw

—3/4 cup of vegetable juice

Fruit group

—1 medium apple, banana, orange, nectarine, or peach

—1/2 cup of chopped, cooked, or canned fruit

—3/4 cup of fruit juice

Milk, yogurt, and cheese group

—1 cup of milk or yogurt

—1 1/2 ounces of natural cheese

—2 ounces of processed cheese

Meat, poultry, fish, dry beans, eggs, and nuts group

—2 to 3 ounces of cooked lean meat, poultry, or fish (1 ounce meat=1/2 cup of cooked dry beans, 1 egg, or 2 tablespoons of peanut butter)

So why not load up with green vegetables, say, and forget everything else? Or eat a bucket of pasta and call it a day? Such an approach might simplify your thinking, but won't do a thing for your nutrition or your sleep. The pyramid does not eliminate any food group; it suggests the right proportion of the different food groups in a healthful diet. Nutritionists recognize some 50 nutrients needed for good health, and no food contains anywhere near that total, so be sure to eat a variety of foods, not just a gargantuan amount of one food.

Notice in the pyramid that fat and sugar (the small circles and triangles) are distributed throughout the food groups, so you'll be getting some even though you cut back on the fats, oils, and sweets group. You need some fat and some cholesterol in your diet. So don't eliminate fat, but do cut back. And giving up eggs? A few years back, some of us were wandering around with a forced smile and a brave front, having given up eggs entirely. It didn't seem natural, and the word today is, have eggs once in awhile, just not a dozen eggs a week (two to four is more like it).

The sense behind all diet now is moderation and variety. Don't overload on anything, whether it be alcohol, salt, red meat, even tofu. Moderation. The world is loaded with diet books and nutrition books. Sleep specialists do recommend proper general diet as a boon to sleep. Check your library or bookstore for a book with the details and sample menus and recipes. Two excellent choices are *60 Days of Low Fat, Low-Cost Meals in Minutes* and *All-American Low-Fat Meals*

> ### Sleeping on eggs ★
>
> Curious about those "egg crate" foam pads you may ★ have seen in hospitals? They work their magic by allowing the body to rest lightly on a series of raised ridges. This allows better circulation than the constant pressure of a flat mattress. The pads may also keep you cool by allowing air to circulate through the indentatations beneath you.
>
> ★

in Minutes, both by M.J. Smith, RD, and published by Chronimed Publishing, Minneapolis.

Sleepy Diet Notes

What's the best bedtime snack? Keep it light. A glass of sparkling water, a cup of herbal tea, a glass of warm milk, Ovaltine, or Horlicks (imported malt drink), with crackers and cheese, just crackers, a slice or two of toast. Experts believe a combination of carbohydrates and protein, such as cheese and crackers, or cereal and milk, is fine at bedtime.

Try to go to bed with a stomach neither full nor empty. A light dinner with protein and carbohydrates is ideal. Remember to count your bedtime snack (and all other snacks) as part of your daily diet if you're watching calories, fat intake, or any other figures.

The bedtime snack of protein and carbohydrate does contain tryptophan, which most specialists see as a possible aid to sleep. Tryptophan,

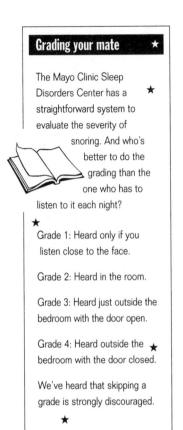

Grading your mate ★

The Mayo Clinic Sleep Disorders Center has a straightforward system to evaluate the severity of snoring. And who's better to do the grading than the one who has to listen to it each night?

Grade 1: Heard only if you listen close to the face.

Grade 2: Heard in the room.

Grade 3: Heard just outside the bedroom with the door open.

Grade 4: Heard outside the bedroom with the door closed.

We've heard that skipping a grade is strongly discouraged.

★

as a natural ingredient in some foods, is converted to serotonin in the brain, and serotonin may make sleep a little easier. However, just as important, many researchers feel, is the strong effect of habit. You get used to having a glass of milk and crackers with cheese at bedtime, you set up yourself to expect them. Same with hot herbal tea, or warm Ovaltine.

Research has shown that a good diet high in carbohydrates and a balance of fat produces a natural elevation of tryptophan. It's probably unwise to depend on your bedtime snack to do this, if your regular diet is deficient. Better to rely on good basic diet, and take a bedtime snack because you like it and like the calming effect.

Good carbohydrate sources are: breads, cereals, grains, fruits, pasta, potatoes, rice, and corn. Good sources of fat are: cheese, cream, ice cream, sour cream, mayo, nuts, and peanut butter. Obviously, there are calorie and other considerations to take into account.

More on Tryptophan

The average person consumes a gram or two of natural tryptophan each day through a regular diet. Tryptophan helps probably half of insomniacs, although its effect is small. Natural tryptophan has been available as a supplement to aid sleep, but was removed from the market in 1989 after reports of side effects in people taking it for an extended period. Some people taking the supplement developed myalgia (aching muscles), with some fatigue and elevated white blood cells (eosinophils). The current government recommendation, and that of most sleep specialists, is to not take supplementary tryptophan. Some point out that the supplements are so much more than a person takes in through food and drink, it makes sense to proceed cautiously.

If you have sleep problems and tryptophan again becomes available, do check with your doctor on what amounts to take, what to eat and what to not eat along with the supplements, and any other recommendations he or she may have.

Melatonin

Melatonin is a chemical produced by the pineal gland in the brain and is thought to have an effect on our sleep-wake rhythm. With a stimulus from darkness, the gland normally secretes melatonin starting at about 9 pm. Blood levels of melatonin rise dramatically, peaking at 2 to 4 am, and returning to the lower daytime levels.

Synthetic melatonin is available, and widespread publicity often creates a rush to health food stores for the hormone. Most scientists, while recognizing that melatonin may reduce the body core temperature and cause drowsiness (although at several hundred times the nighttime peak levels the body produces), caution against use of synthetic melatonin to combat insomnia.

The hormone is promising, but medical studies have been carried out primarily on laboratory animals; studies on humans are being done and more studies are needed to determine proper dosage, side effects, what conditions preclude its use—such as pregnancy and autoimmune disorders— what time of day the dose should be taken, and many other considerations.

Sleep specialists caution that synthetic melatonin is a hormone, not a dietary supplement, and warn against unrestricted use, especially in older people.

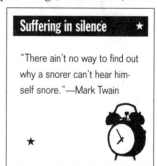

Suffering in silence ★

"There ain't no way to find out why a snorer can't hear himself snore."—Mark Twain

★

Most specialists acknowledge that melatonin is very promising as part of the treatment of insomnia, and may help many poor sleepers. But they urge caution until the proper studies have been completed, and not to look forward to a single pill to alleviate insomnia as aspirin often alleviates a headache.

Complex Carbs

Try to return to Grandma's kitchen, or at least to Grandma's ingredients. In her day, there was little choice, but today you have to search out the unrefined flour, the unrefined rice, the unrefined anything. We're surrounded by refined foods, so treated to keep longer on the supermarket shelves—and for no other reason. Any plant food is a carbohydrate—a complex carbohydrate in its natural state. Only after these grains, sugars, and other carbs have been refined—denuded of their fiber and nutrients—are they called refined or simple carbohydrates. Avoid the simple, refined carbs; go for the complex and unrefined.

Minerals and Vitamins

Magnesium and calcium are natural sedatives, and they do help some people sleep better. Stress, of course, depletes the body's calcium and magnesium, our natural relaxants. If this is a problem, some specialists recommend two parts calcium to one part magnesium—800 mg calcium and 400 mg magnesium for adults, 1200 mg calcium with 600 mg magnesium for teenagers and pregnant women. Some experts advise giving equal amounts of both minerals.

A well-rounded diet is the best source of vitamins, but additional vitamins sometimes help with sleep. Individuals react quite differently to vitamin supplements, so don't use them without thinking—tossing down a handful of vitamin pills on the run is not recommended.

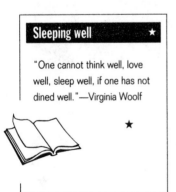

Sleeping well ★

"One cannot think well, love well, sleep well, if one has not dined well."—Virginia Woolf

★

The B complex vitamins are important in regulating your body's production of serotonin. Vitamin B3 (niacin) has been shown to help some people who have depression along with insomnia. Some 50 to 100 mg per day of B3 may increase tryptophan production and help with mild depression as well as the accompanying insomnia.

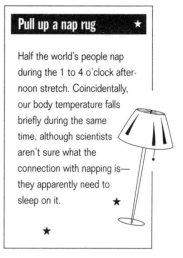

Pull up a nap rug ★

Half the world's people nap during the 1 to 4 o'clock afternoon stretch. Coincidentally, our body temperature falls briefly during the same time, although scientists aren't sure what the connection with napping is— they apparently need to sleep on it. ★

★

Vitamin B12 and folic acid, another part of the vitamin B family, also have been shown to promote sleep in some people. The most sensible recommendation about vitamin intake to help with your sleep problems is try a course of the B complex multivitamin supplement instead of trying individual B vitamins. The B complex is available with either 50 mg or 100 mg of each B vitamin. Take one supplement a day for possible help. But do monitor your results. A few people react adversely to B vitamins; the supplement excites them and promotes sleeplessness.

When you try mineral or vitamin supplements, do so in a reasonable dosage and don't expect instant results. Try the supplement over a week or two and note its effects. The changes should be subtle, and may help you get better sleep—along with an overall sleep plan of diet, exercise, relaxation, and the like.

Herbs

Certain herbs are widely prescribed by herbalists to help you fall asleep and stay asleep. Valerian is well known for its sedative and sleep inducing properties, especially if you have problems with anxiety, muscle fatigue, stress. Take it as a bedtime tea with honey, and sip it leisurely during a hot bath or while preparing for bed. While some are available in pill form, these other herbs also are often helpful (and not harmful) when sipped as tea: primrose, lemon balm, chamomile, passion flower, catnip, and hops.

Results can be good to excellent, but herbs are not foolproof. Take the advice of an herbalist, go with a low dose, and try the teas first.

Chapter 9

Exercise & Relaxation

Let's not get uptight over relaxation . . . or exercise. So much has been written and rebutted about how and why to keep in shape that it's easy to get lost in the cross-currents and drop the whole subject.

Don't lose your way. We're not talking about full-time training for the Olympics, we're talking about some pleasant (if possible) exercise and a few relaxation ideas to help shrug off tension and stay loose. And the ideas have to work for you, not someone else much younger and in far better shape. Pick exercise and relaxation tips that make sense for you and try them. Keep the ones that work, and let them become habitual. You'll discover, over time, that you're probably sleeping better and feeling better physically and emotionally.

And it costs nothing. Oh, you can spend a wad on exercise equipment, high-dollar spandex togs, fitness club memberships. But you don't have to. Good walking shoes are important, but everything else is optional. What does it cost to take a walk? And that's one of the few exercises that all authorities agree on—regular brisk walking.

So, deep breathe and read on. Why exercise? Is there truly a benefit from regular exercise? Mark Twain, after all, said he never exercised when he could avoid it, because he "never could see any advantage in being tired." As a lifetime fan of Twain, and an individual predisposed to sitting rather than moving about, I have to take issue, much as it hurts.

Make up your mind ★

Each year, Americans spend more than $98 million on ★ over-the-counter remedies to help them sleep at night, and another $50 million on caffeine tablets to help them stay awake during the day. ★

There is a big advantage in being tired at the end of the day, at bedtime: You may sleep better. Not only that, you'll feel more refreshed. As a late-comer to exercise—and mild, at that—I can attest to the benefits. Don't make the mistakes I did, and expect instant results. A brisk walk of half an hour doesn't guarantee you better sleep for that night. But a habit of three or more such brisk walks each week nearly always results in generally better sleep and better shape. And it's never too late to start. Here are a few reasons:

- Regular exercise over time may not only facilitate sleep, but also will improve your circulation, help build stronger bones (more resistive to osteoarthritis), lower your blood pressure, help you shed extra pounds, give you better muscle tone.

- None of this happens overnight, so regularity is the key, even if it's a few exercise times per week.

> ### Bathing beauty ★
>
> It is thought that the body begins to get drowsy as its temperature drops. A warm bath 4 or 5 hours before bedtime will raise your temperature. Then, as it begins to fall, you'll feel more tired, making it easier to fall asleep.

- The fatigue produced by exercise has been called the best tranquilizer in the world.

- Studies have shown that exercise not only promotes sleep, but tends to promote better sleep—that is, sleep with more deep restorative sleep and somewhat less REM sleep. Other studies confirm that physically fit people such as athletes in training do have a larger percentage of their sleep as deep delta.

- And regular exercise contributes to an overall sense of feeling good, of being (dare we say it?) happier. If you're a lifetime professional grouch, maybe you can resist. And if you are seriously depressed, you'll still benefit from good exercise, but probably not to the extent of feeling happy, at least early in the exercise program. Otherwise, the good feelings are hard to resist.

- Muscle tone and strength will increase over time only after exercise, when they are at rest and rebuilding. A muscle seldom used is not undergoing improvement.

- If you do not move through at least mild exercise, your circulation and breathing get sluggish, you build up tension, you have energy not being used which puts your nervous system at fast idle with muscles aching to move.

- Exercise activates some endocrine glands, charges your body with more vitality, and provides a natural way to help prevent the negative effects of stress.

- Epinephrine, the body hormone that stimulates endorphins, your natural tranquilizers, is said to double in the body after just 10 to 15 minutes of sustained exercise. For long-lasting effects from increased endorphins, make your exercise regular.

- With a mild exercise program, especially if you're essentially sedentary, begin to look for some improvement in 3 or 4 weeks. By then, with regular exercise, most people will be more relaxed, less tense than before, and generally sleeping better. Results are not instant, but they do occur if we stay with the exercise.

The Temperature Connection

Your body temperature has a lot to do with good sleep, specialists are discovering. Body temperature typically peaks in late afternoon or early evening between 7 and 9, then drops before sleep onset and drops faster immediately after you fall asleep. Body temperature then drops to its lowest around 4 to 6 am, and starts to rise as you wake up. The variation between highs and lows is about 2 degrees F.

So, any exercise that raises your body temperature some 2 degrees for about 20 minutes can affect how readily you fall asleep. And a falling body temperature is strongly associated with falling asleep. In people with insomnia, the body temperature remains significantly higher at night than it does in those who sleep well.

If you increase body temperature through exercise about 5 or 6 hours before going to bed, your temperature generally will drop about the time you want to go to sleep and may increase your chances of falling asleep with few problems. That usually means exercising around 5 or 6 in the afternoon. While most specialists agree that this is the best time to let exercise help your sleep, they recognize that it may be impossible for some of us. We may have to exercise in the morning or at noon.

Another way to take advantage of the temperature connection is by taking a hot bath in the evening. A hot bath anytime helps you relax as you cool down, and in the evening may aid falling asleep.

Which Exercises for You?

There's no perfect exercise, and what works for you may not work for your friends. But pick and choose, using the following guidelines:

- Age (in general terms). Many people find that, even with moderate exercise, they begin to notice changes after about age 35 to 40, with gravity taking its toll and pounds mounting. It's always easier to keep fit than to get fit once you're in less than top shape.

- Are you in bad shape? An aging couch potato, along with many of us? It's a good idea to check with your doctor before starting exercises, then pick one or two and start gradually. It makes no sense to propel yourself from the couch to a furious jogging routine—your body will rebel. Easy does it.

- With any exercise, especially if you're just beginning, watch for signs like tightness in the chest, dizziness, gasping for breath, upset stomach. If you experience anything like this, stop and rest. If it continues, call your doctor.

- Set your goal by your heart rate. For aerobic exercising, find your maximum heart rate by subtracting your age (say you're 45) from 220. Then figure 60 to 75 percent of that as your target heart rate: 220-45= 175 X .60=105. 175 X .75= 130 (rounded). So your target heart rate is a pulse of 105 to 130 per minute. If you've exercised with regularity, you know how to quick check your pulse as you work out: take your pulse for 10 seconds and multiply by 6.

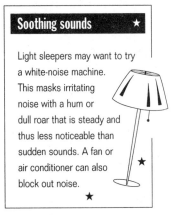

Soothing sounds ★

Light sleepers may want to try a white-noise machine. This masks irritating noise with a hum or dull roar that is steady and thus less noticeable than sudden sounds. A fan or air conditioner can also block out noise.

- You may want to check your target zone on the accompanying chart. If you're just beginning and don't want to check things as you work out, exercise until you're a little breathless, and have worked up a bit of a sweat. Over 10 to 20 minutes, that's about right, then cool down.

Exercise Target Zone
(beats per minute)

Age	Beats per minute
20	120-150
25	117-146
30	114-142
35	111-138
40	108-135
45	105-131
50	102-127
55	99-123
60	96-120
65	93-116
70	90-113

- With any exercise, warm up first. Go through the routine in slow motion and stretch and bend to limber up for 5 minutes or so. Then get into the exercise routine for about 20 minutes, and cool down (by slowing down, walking slower, finally stopping) for another 5 minutes. That's a half hour that can do wonders if you stick with it and work up gradually to your target heart rate.

- Consider exercises you're going to enjoy, or at least not detest, because it just makes sense to do things you like, and increases your chance of staying with it.

- Remember, there are three kinds of exercise: Aerobic (walking, biking, swimming, and more) helps improve cardiovascular fitness. Strength training (weight lifting, some calisthenics, chopping wood) helps improve muscle fitness and fight fatigue. Flexibility exercise (stretching and bending, recommended as part of your warm-up) develops and maintains good range of motion in your joints and muscles.

Can you learn in your sleep? ★

Subliminal tapes. Ah yes, you've seen the ads—learn a second language or solve life's problems with the help of a whispered, tape recorded message that plays as you sleep. One problem, though: They don't work. Plus, they can interfere with the deep, restorative stages of sleep. ★

Walking

If forced to pick one form of exercise over all others, many specialists would go with walking. You don't have to learn a new skill to do it, walking is safe, walking is aerobic, and it can be done alone, with a friend, or with a group. In rotten weather, too cold or rainy for an outdoor walk, many people use a local mall. Check yours and you're likely to find it open early for walkers during the winter months.

We are not talking about strolling, although that's a most pleasant way to spend time too. No, we're talking about brisk walking. How fast? Marching right along and swinging your arms vigorously. If you find yourself breathing deeply and beginning to sweat after 10 minutes of walking, you're going at a good pace.

Some people like to walk to music, and headphones become as important as shoes. Others like to talk with a friend while walking at a brisk pace, which is another good measurement. If you can still carry on a conversation while walking fast, you're not going too fast.

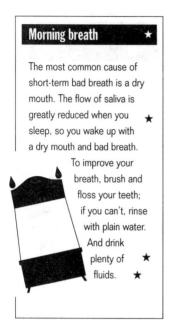

Morning breath ★

The most common cause of short-term bad breath is a dry mouth. The flow of saliva is greatly reduced when you ★ sleep, so you wake up with a dry mouth and bad breath. To improve your breath, brush and floss your teeth; if you can't, rinse with plain water. And drink plenty of ★ fluids. ★

One important hint about walking: take a stick along, or a cane, or a rolled up umbrella. Not for protection, but to get out of the robot-like sameness of walking. Swing the stick around, knock the heads off some dandelions, force yourself to turn and bend a bit. It will keep you from getting cramped muscles. Walking with your dog will help both of you (depending on the mood of the dog).

And walking over a rough surface rather than sidewalk is even better if you can do it. A hike over a meadow, over the grasses of a park, through the woods—all are more beneficial than on a clear sidewalk, albeit hard to find for some of us. Just make sure to be careful of your footing.

Other Aerobics

Jogging is still popular and if you want to get into it, check with jogger friends, your local "Y" or other sources. Jogging of course is hard impact, and may be more than most middle age people want.

The stationary bike is another choice. Judging from the number found at garage sales, it may be difficult to keep doing, but it does have the advantage of being available, good weather or bad.

Regular biking is fine if you like it. Some people alternate stationary and regular biking. For more of a challenge, look into mountain bikes. Don't forget dancing as a good aerobic workout. It can be fun, involve you in a group, and provide aerobic exercise too. And it may help you loosen up as well as work out.

Then there are swimming, skating, cross-country skiing, you name it. And some of us find it pays to sign up with a community aerobics class, often through the "Y". For middle age and older, probably the low-impact aerobics is best, with monitoring of pulse and good warm-ups and cool-downs. This offers a structure and deadlines (which some of us need): three or four or five times a week, morning or evening, pay in advance but not a fortune, and hope for an enthusiastic leader.

And remember, exercise specialists advise putting more effort into our daily tasks. Park away from the office, or in the far corner of the parking lot and walk. Hike between floors rather than use the elevators. Toss your remote TV control so you have to get up to change channels. Many of us, however, have had little luck with this approach, and find we need more planned exercise time.

A fine way to get as much of a workout as you need, maybe more, is to spend some time babysitting a grandchild, says Dr. Robert S. Eliot, author of *From Stress to Strength*, and I concur.

Rather than spend hours and big bucks studying various exercise programs and hardware, just do it. And keep on doing it. Two times to avoid vigorous exercise: No closer to bedtime than 4 to 6 hours before, or your body will be too invigorated for sleep. And, right after a big meal.

Relaxation Strategies

Yes, relaxation techniques can be vital to improving your sleep. And no, not everyone likes them, not everyone can do them the first time, and not everyone needs them.

But most of us do. You'll find a wealth of material on relaxation techniques at your library or bookstore, or your local video stores. Also, check your local "Y" or adult education classes; you're likely to find enough relaxation techniques to make your head swim (which doesn't help). Here are a few basic techniques that have proven very helpful to most people.

Progressive Muscle Relaxation

This is for anyone, and is especially good for those of us who have trouble relaxing, or are just getting started. The exercise itself gives you a good idea of where your tension is, even though you may not be aware of it.

Try this basic relaxation in the evening, at bedtime, even in bed:

1. Choose a quiet, comfortable place.

2. Loosen tight clothing and take off your shoes (if in bed for the night, presumably you're in your pajamas or the altogether).

3. Lie as comfortably as you can and close your eyes if you wish, uncross your legs, and rest your hands flat with palms up.

4. Now, with each of the following areas, first tense your muscles, then relax and let go. The difference shows you what tenseness is, and a released tense muscle naturally relaxes momentarily. Try to prolong it. With each area, tense as much as you can; really work at it, for a count of 10. Breathe deeply and feel the tension, then let the tension go as you breathe out, and feel the relaxation. Take time to feel the difference; this is the strength of progressive relaxation.

Toes—
Curl your toes toward you, and tighten your instep. And relax.

Calves—
Point your toes, your whole feet, toward your face. Tighten those ankle and calf muscles. Really do it! And relax.

Buttocks—
Push your buttocks hard against the bed or floor and make your body feel heavy. Squeeze your gluteals. And relax.

Hands and forearms—
Make tight fists (better when you hold your arms a few inches off the surface), and tighten arm muscles like holding a heavy iron bar. Drop your arms and relax.

Abdomen—
Tense your abdomen as though you expect a punch in the stomach.
And relax.

Shoulders—
Shrug your shoulders as high as you can, way up toward your ears!
And relax.

Throat—
With your chin, press your throat down hard. And relax.

Neck and head—
Press your neck and head back and up, against the backs of your
shoulders, stretching your neck. And relax.

Face—
Have some fun with this. Tighten as many facial muscles as you can,
including your forehead, eyes, jaw, cheeks, chin, nose. Make a wild
grimace. And relax.

And that's it. You may have trouble isolating these areas at first, but stay
with it until you feel the progressive relaxation.

The procedure should take 15 to 20 minutes. If you haven't the time,
try this shortened version (you can do it sitting on a plane, in your
office, almost anywhere):

1. Tighten and tense the whole upper part of your body.

2. Suck in your abdomen and tense your buttocks.

3. Try to force your body off the chair by pressing the soles of your feet
   hard against the floor and using your calf and other leg muscles.

Abdominal Breathing

This is another basic technique that works for most people:

1. Lie on your back, loosen clothing, and try to relax.

2. Forget everything you ever learned about standing at attention, suck-
   ing that abdomen in, breathing with heaving chests.

3. Observe closely. See how you breathe when you're not forcing it at all. You will be breathing with your abdomen, which is good.

4. Place your hands on your abdomen and chest and feel the difference in breathing.

5. Place your hands over your abdomen with fingertips touching and see how they move apart as you breathe. Try stretching your arms over your head. This helps stop chest breathing and lets you feel the abdomen breathing first, then the chest.

6. Try to feel this deep abdominal breathing by inhaling to a count of six, then exhaling to a reverse count, emptying your lungs. Breathe in through your nose and out through your nose or mouth.

This deep breathing technique does take a little practice, but it is well worth it, and not that difficult. Once you feel it, you have it. A period of deep abdominal breathing can take the edge off nearly any tension and often provides the relaxation you need for falling asleep, and staying asleep.

Meditation

The many forms of meditation may work for you, but selection is an individual matter. Yoga, transcendental meditation (concentrating on a mantra, or quieting word), mental imagery (imagining yourself on a secluded tropical beach . . . .) and countless other meditative approaches are worth exploring.

All are designed to provide an inner peace, slow down the body functions like breathing and heart rate, and focus you on sensations of calm. Finding the ones best for you will take some trying. However, getting a good grasp on progressive muscle relaxation and deep abdominal breathing, as outlined above, will help in themselves and will help you find additional techniques if you want to.

I've had good results with one yoga maneuver recommended by Dale L. Anderson, MD: alternate nostril breathing. It's a quiet form of stress relief and takes little space:

- Sit on the floor or in bed in the lotus position (erect with knees bent and ankles crossed) or just your back straight. Close your eyes and mouth.

- Close your right nostril by pressing with your right thumb. Keep your other fingers bent as though you were going to pinch your nose. Breathe in through the left nostril, comfortably filling your lungs but not forcing it.

- Close your nose for a few seconds by gently squeezing.

- Release the right nostril and exhale slowly. Then breathe in through the right nostril to fill the lungs. Again close the nose, this time by reapplying the thumb. Then release your left nostril, breathe out slowly, and begin again.

- Repeat the whole sequence five times or more. Stop if you get dizzy, which may happen at first. And use relaxed breathing, that causes no noise in or out. This simple little procedure lets you—forces you—to concentrate on the breathing and many find it a good way to totally relax for sleep.

Are Naps Beneficial? Yes! (and No)

First, the No: If you have serious insomnia, with your sleep cycle way out of kilter, don't nap during the day. It will only cause more trouble. Also, if you're middle age or older, resist the naps if you're trying to sleep longer at night.

Otherwise, welcome the nap as one of nature's marvelous ways of relaxing and refreshing you. Sleep specialists have been

"Cutting" out snoring ★

Snoring affects about half of men and 30 percent of women—most age 50 or older. Snoring occurs when air flows past relaxed tissues as you breathe. The sagging tissues narrow your airway, causing the tissues to flutter. Losing weight or changing sleep positions may help, but laser surgery is also an alternative for some. Laser surgery trims the soft palate and uvula (that triangular piece of tissue hanging in the back of your mouth), reducing the amount ★ of vibrating tissue. ★

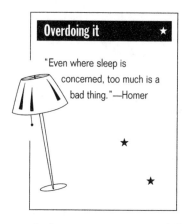

Overdoing it ★

"Even where sleep is concerned, too much is a bad thing." —Homer

★

★

ambivalent about naps, but most now see them as beneficial and part of a normal sleep-wake pattern. It's one of the most welcome blessings they've bestowed, to those of us who know the beauties of a nap, whether or not we can work them in.

And that includes nearly everyone. We've been trapped in monophasic guidelines for too long—that we are creatures of the day and night, with no cheating by slipping in naps.

As it turns out, most specialists feel, we're biphasic, with our days broken into two phases of diminished alertness—nocturnal and midafternoon.

Isn't it amazing how we get sleepy in early or midafternoon following a big lunch? No, say the specialists, it's not. We tend to feel the need for some sleep about 8 hours after we get up, lunch or no lunch. In fact, say the specialists, most people will take a nap during the day whenever they have a chance, meals or no meals; students and retirees take more naps because they have more opportunities. (There are conservatives among us—me, for instance—who feel that a large lunch at least contributes to feeling sleepy in early afternoon, but we're not about to foresake lunch to prove it.)

An afternoon nap can be a wonderfully effective tool for catching up on your sleep debt. Watch the length, though. Most sleep experts agree that you'll feel groggy for 5 to 15 minutes after a nap, called "sleep inertia." They point out that the temporary inconvenience is more than offset by improved alertness and a buoyed mood. And a nap will do more for you than a similar period of sleep tacked onto your morning sleep.

Take a nap at any time you feel the need, and have the opportunity, but realize that you'll get the best return on your investment if that nap is some 8 hours after your morning awakening, and some 8 hours before your bedtime.

For best results, take short naps of no more than 30 minutes (10 to 15 minutes will refresh you) or naps of 2 hours or more. Nothing in between. Anything in between is likely to leave you with pronounced sleep inertia on awakening. Naps of 2 hours or more (pretty rare, but delightful) need to be planned, since they will affect your nighttime sleep. For a quick, short nap, relax in an easy chair and hold a spoon over the chair arm with an empty metal pie plate beneath it. By the time you sleep enough for the spoon to slip from your fingers and bang the pan, you'll have an adequate nap and feel refreshed. At least Salvador Dali used that method. Feel free to develop your own.

By the way, don't try to nap if you are not sleepy. The only exception here is an occasional rest prophylactically when you know you're going to have a busy, sleep-deprived night ahead (travel, banquet, graduation party, etc.).

Chapter 10

The Limited Role of
Sleeping Pills

Many sleep specialists advise never taking pills for sleep, period. A few doctors may still prescribe them freely. And perhaps the majority prescribe sleeping pills (hypnotics) for brief periods under specific situations, with extreme caution. Take care if you use hypnotics. Be sure you and your physician have good reasons for it, and personally, be sure you have the strength and determination to use them just occasionally. Taking hypnotics is easy; stopping can be difficult, even after a short time.

There's no question that natural sleep is best, achieved by good sleep hygiene, diet, exercise, relaxation techniques, and the like.

There's also no question that sleeping medications have been vastly overused, treating insomnia—a symptom in itself—and masking the underlying cause. This occurred more often in the 1960s with use of barbiturates, less so in recent years with the benzodiazepines.

The two big problems with using sleeping pills for insomnia: (1) habituation, (2) rebound effect.

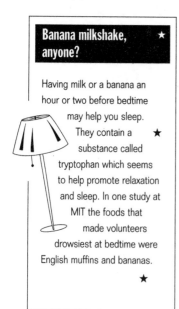

Banana milkshake, anyone? ★

Having milk or a banana an hour or two before bedtime may help you sleep. They contain a ★ substance called tryptophan which seems to help promote relaxation and sleep. In one study at MIT the foods that made volunteers drowsiest at bedtime were English muffins and bananas.

★

In other words, there is always a potential for becoming dependent on the sleeping pill effect, especially if you've had other addictive reactions to, say, cigarettes, drinking, or gambling. Withdrawal from hypnotics is likely to be uncomfortable.

Even if you take a hypnotic for two or three nights, when you stop, your insomnia will be as bad as before, if not worse. This is the rather gloomy but realistic advice from most sleep specialists. Yes, there are specific times when sleeping pills are called for. No, the pills will not solve your insomnia, but just help get you past a particularly rough time, and after stopping, you'll still need to deal with your insomnia.

When Sleeping Pills May Be Used

With caution, hypnotics may be indicated for:

- Short-term insomnia with known cause, such as jet lag for a night or two.

- Acute insomnia for occasional severe stress, such as for a night or two after witnessing a traumatic accident or suffering loss of a friend or loved one.

- Prophylactically, such as for a night before a presentation that has you wide awake, as it has in the past. If used this way, it should be the only such pill you take that week.

- In dramatic changes of sleep environment such as undergoing a change of night shift, to aid adaptation. Hypnotics do not speed the adaptation, but may help you get to sleep for the first 2 or 3 days.

> ### Skip the nightly news ★
>
> You may want to consider ★ skipping the 10 o'clock news. It's full of stories about the latest war, murder, robbery, and accident, which do nothing to act as a sleep-inducing lullaby. Instead, laugh with a good book or watch a TV comedy.
>
> ★

One sleep specialist, very conservative in prescribing pills for sleep, does so with confidence for this patient: A professional woman drives across two states for a long weekend with her mother, and does so every summer. The relationship has been tenuous for years, and she asks for sleeping pills to help her before and during the visit. He prescribes 10 pills, she immediately feels better just having them (the placebo effect sometimes helps without ever taking the pills), and the next year she comes in with the same request. She also has eight of the previous pills left. No question, he says, this patient benefits and is not likely to have withdrawal problems, not at two pills a year.

That's an extreme example, but a good one to keep in mind. You can take charge of your sleep problems and solutions. Do all the nonprescription things you can, to assure good sleep. And regard sleeping pills with caution.

If your doctor does prescribe them, be sure you follow directions. Don't double up on them, never drink alcohol when you're taking sleeping pills, and remember that older people react more strongly in general.

When Sleeping Pills Should Not Be Used

Sleeping pills are usually not prescribed in these situations:

- When you have not talked about medications with your doctor. Sleeping pills can interact with other drugs, including nonprescription medicines, so be sure your doctor knows all the medications you're taking.

- When you have sleep apnea or strong indications of it. Many sleeping pills are respiratory depressants, and can worsen apnea or other respiratory situations.

- When you have chronic insomnia, lasting 6 months or more. Sleeping pills are of little value in such cases, except to ease poor sleepers through periodic flare-ups. The treatment must center on the underlying cause.

- When you are taking other mood-altering drugs; be sure your doctor knows this. Physicians are careful about drug interactions, but since we sometimes have prescriptions from different doctors, as well as nonprescription medications, it's wise to be sure and remind your doctor about all you're taking.

- When you are pregnant, or think you may be. Discuss this with your doctor.

Which Sleeping Pills?

Go with your doctor's recommendations, and feel free to ask him or her about possible side effects, what to look for, and precise dose instructions. It sometimes helps to question your pharmacist too, if you're not clear.

Also, any so-called sleeping pills you may buy without a prescription, such as Sominex and Nytol, have antihistamine as the main ingredient. Histamine is the chemical released when tissues are irritated, contributing to itching, asthma, hay fever, and other allergies. Antihistamines are designed to counter these effects and one common side effect is drowsiness. Check with your physician before regular use of medications containing antihistamine.

Earlier, barbiturates were used extensively but most sleeping medications—hypnotics—used today are benzodiazepines, the "valium-like" drugs. Benzodiazepines were introduced in 1960 with chlordiazepoxide (Librium), shortly followed by diazepam (Valium) and in 1970, flurazepam (Dalmane), the first benzodiazepine specifically recommended for sleep.

In the 1980s, other shorter acting benzodiazepines such as temazepam (Restoril) and triazolam (Halcion) were introduced.

Other non-benzodiazepines such as zolpidem (Ambien) have been introduced, and these, along with some remaining use of barbiturates, gives a wide variety of medications available. Talk them over with your doctor if he or she prescribes one. Generally, shorter acting drugs are preferred—those with shorter half-life. The half-life of a drug is the time it take for 50 percent of it to disappear from your bloodstream.

Short half-life usually means less carry-over drug effect on the next day. If your doctor wants that effect—if you are particularly anxious or ill, for example—he or she may choose a sleeping medication with a longer half-life.

Hypnotics are potent medications with side effects and dramatic results. Rather than trying to memorize the side effects, ask your doctor and be sure you know what to expect. Just as important, be sure you take the medication as directed and report any ill effects.

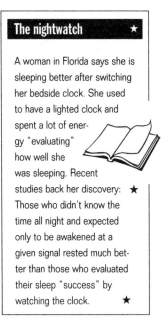

The nightwatch ★

A woman in Florida says she is sleeping better after switching her bedside clock. She used to have a lighted clock and spent a lot of energy "evaluating" how well she was sleeping. Recent studies back her discovery: ★ Those who didn't know the time all night and expected only to be awakened at a given signal rested much better than those who evaluated their sleep "success" by watching the clock. ★

Chapter 11

Pursuing Traveling Sleep

So you're traveling more in your work, and enjoying it less? Taking vacations and feeling dragged out? Getting a good night's sleep on the road is not all that difficult, but it does require planning. It's worth it. On a business trip, you'll appreciate the good rest and feeling refreshed. On a vacation, you'll enjoy it more if you maintain your good sleep habits.

The Anderson Approach

One of the most innovative advisors on how to get good sleep while traveling is Dale L. Anderson, MD, of Minneapolis, who spends a great deal of time traveling himself. He's a nationally recognized speaker, humorist, and relaxation consultant. (See Chapter 7: Exercise and Relaxation.) When he travels, he remembers the little things:

Everyone can handle a certain number of adverse factors involving time schedules, missed connecting flights, poor food, jet lag, and so many more. But it may take just one more to break the camel's back, so pay attention to little things. "A tired body, physically and mentally, does not allow the normal mechanisms to fight stress and illness. The key is getting proper rest and sleep." How? By paying attention to the little things:

- Avoid caffeine at least 6 hours before bedtime (coffee, tea, cola or other caffeine-containing soft drinks and unnecessary medications)

- Avoid chocolate (including that complimentary chocolate on your hotel pillow)

- Avoid nasal sprays

- Avoid smoking. Nicotine is a stimulant.

- Avoid alcohol

- Avoid high sugar intake at bedtime

- Avoid sodium

- Avoid late dinners, large dinners

- Avoid dehydration (environmental and within the body)

- Avoid exercising too close to bedtime. This raises body metabolism for several hours, making it more difficult to slow the body down for sleep.

- Avoid clock watching. People with lighted clocks at bedside spend a significant amount of time checking it to see how they're doing. Those who don't know what time it is generally sleep better.

- Avoid watching evening news on television. The usual 10 o'clock news is not 'user friendly,' but is filled with accidents, violent crime, catastrophes—not sleep-inducing.

A discouraging list? Perhaps, but sleepless nights on the road can be more than discouraging. And few of us will adhere to all of Dr. Anderson's guidelines. To balance your approach, here are several things for you to do for a good night's sleep while traveling:

Sleepwalking myths ★

Not too long ago, medical schools were teaching their students that if sleepwalking continued through adolescence and into adulthood, a strong likelihood of a psychiatric disorder existed. It's simply not true. Sleepwalking can be perfectly normal, whatever your age. If a family member is a nocturnal roamer, don't wake them up. No, not because they'll go crazy or get lockjaw or any number of other myths. There's simply no reason to rouse them. Just guide your sleepwalker safely and gently to bed. ★

- Raise your endorphins. This reduces pain, relaxes muscles, suppresses the appetite, and creates a good feeling of optimism and happiness. Do it by:

—Taking a hot bath

—Making friendly connections by calling home, looking at family pictures, saying a prayer.

—Laughing with a good book or watching TV comedy

—Physical conditioning (up to within 4 to 6 hours before bedtime)

- Rearrange your hotel room. Most accidents in a strange room are from falling or tripping over furniture or "travel debris." Move the telephone, clock radio, and other essentials close to the bed so you will not injure yourself in a groping lunge during the night or on awakening.

- Bring nightlights. They're not just for kids. Plug them in so you can navigate the room without turning on a bright light.

- Request a different pillow if yours is not right. Often hotel management will provide a more comfortable one. If you have a special pillow that nearly always assures sleep, bring it along. Dr. Anderson brings his own.

- Raise the head of the bed by placing pillows under the mattress if you habitually have heartburn (and avoid heavy, spicy meals).

- Control noise by:

—Reserving a room on the tenth floor or above if on the street side of the hotel

—Getting a room away from elevators or stairways, vending or ice machines, and likely party rooms such as hospitality suites. Let the desk know if noise is disruptive.

—Using soft ear plugs

—Requesting a small electric fan or using the air conditioner to provide some air movement and a hum to mask outside noise

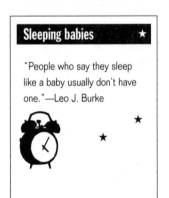

Sleeping babies ★

"People who say they sleep like a baby usually don't have one."—Leo J. Burke

- Get a room with east or south exposure for more morning sun, making it easier to wake up in the morning. If south of the equator, get a room with east or north exposure.

- Keep the room at 65 degrees in the afternoon and night. Check it as soon as you arrive and call management if there is a problem.

Dr. Anderson's advice appears in *The Business Traveler's Guide to Good Health on the Road*, edited by Karl Neumann, MD, and Maury Rosenbaum, Chronimed Publishing, Minneapolis, MN 1994.

Exercises for the Traveler

If traveling by car, some easy exercises along the way will help you relieve stress and sleep better at night. Stuck in a traffic jam? Strengthen your pectorals by putting your hands together as if praying, with wrists in front of your forehead. Press hands together hard, but for no longer than a second or two. You'll feel the strain in your chest muscles (pecs). Repeat with hands the same or move them up and down in front of your chest and head, while doing 1-second contractions.

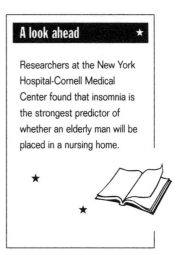

A look ahead ★

Researchers at the New York Hospital-Cornell Medical Center found that insomnia is the strongest predictor of whether an elderly man will be placed in a nursing home.

Another simple exercise begins with elbows at your waist, extended or bent. Then press your arms forcefully against your sides. You can do this side squeezing wherever you are.

Another variation that can be done anywhere: Put your elbows against the back of your chair or wall and push, or put both palms directly over your navel and push.

For neck muscles, where we often get troubling tenseness, exaggerate a shoulder shrug, bring shoulders forward, raise them as high as you can, then push them back and down. Shoulder shrugs are great for reducing tension.

For your front and side neck muscles, put your palms, fingers pointing upward, on your forehead and apply resistance as you slowly flex your head forward. Do only three repetitions if you haven't exercised the neck before. Then, lock your fingers and place palms on the back of your head, and apply resistance. Don't extend your head to the rear. Then

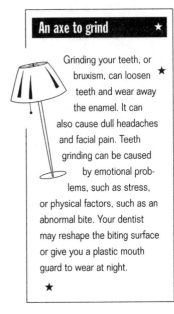

An axe to grind ★

Grinding your teeth, or bruxism, can loosen ★ teeth and wear away the enamel. It can also cause dull headaches and facial pain. Teeth grinding can be caused by emotional problems, such as stress, or physical factors, such as an abnormal bite. Your dentist may reshape the biting surface or give you a plastic mouth guard to wear at night.

★

place your right palm against the side of your head above the ear, flex your head to the right against resistance, and do the same on the left.

If you're prone to headaches, perhaps it's better not to apply resistance to head movement. Instead, just lower your head forward slowly and let it hang for 10 to 20 seconds. Do this three times.

In a plane, seat exercises are good. British Airways offers these suggestions for keeping fit while you sit:

Hands—Rotate your wrists clockwise and reverse.

• Shake your hands out.

Neck—Rotate your neck slowly five times each way.

• Raise shoulders, breathe out, drop, 4 or 5 times.

• Rotate shoulders backward 5 times, forward 5.

• Turn to the back of your seat, keeping hips square, 3 to 5 times.

Head—With fingertips, lightly massage from temple to jaw.

• Rest your head forward on your thumbs, squeeze along eyebrows with thumb and forefinger.

• Massage along upper jaw, then lower jaw.

Ankles—Rotate your ankles 10 times clockwise, then 10 times counterclockwise.

• With feet on the floor, raise your heels, then relax. Repeat 20 to 30 times.

When You Arrive

On arrival, walking is one of the best exercises to relax and help you adjust. Be sure to take good walking shoes. And of course check out where to walk with hotel management, to be sure you're in safe territory. If there's any question, or if the weather is awful, walk in place in your room. To walk in place and benefit, lift your knees high and vigorously pump your arms back and forth. Move slightly forward, backward, or to the side, for variety.

Other simple exercises you can do in your hotel room or bedroom, to promote well being and good sleep:

Lunges, to work muscles in front of the thighs. Hands on hips, keeping upper body erect, step forward with one foot. First, a few inches in front of the stationary foot, and with each step a little further. Go as far with the lunge as is comfortable, perhaps 8 to 10 lunges.

Kneebends are excellent. Hold onto a surface for balance if you want and don't squat below a 90-degree angle at the knees or you might injure the knee ligaments. Keep hips tucked under, to avoid back pain. Look up and keep your chest high.

Rising on balls of your feet will strengthen your calves. You can do this standing in line, too.

For hamstring muscles at the back of the thigh, stand erect and lift one foot. This causes the knee to bend, but don't let it go forward. Keep it next to the other knee or even back of it as you stretch; you'll feel it. Do this exercise slowly.

To work the gluteals, extend your leg to the rear, lunges or knee bends, walking upstairs.

Many hotels and motels offer pools, whirlpools, workout rooms, a variety of exercise options. On a tight schedule, you may not have time for a full workout, or need it.

Chapter 12

Sleep Disorders,
Parasomnias, et al.

We wind up with a look at sleep disorders and parasomnias. These include some of the more bizarre conditions that can cause sleep loss or poor sleep quality and very often excessive daytime sleepiness.

Sleep researchers have identified some 84 disorders of the sleep-wake state that can result in poor health, poor quality of life, and even safety. Some problems with staying awake, staying on a schedule, keeping alert, do contribute to accidents. More often, some of the 84 can make your life miserable.

Fortunately, sleep disorders—actual disorders of your sleep process that are active during sleep and often not active when you are awake—are relatively rare. And sleep specialists have found ways to eliminate or control many such conditions.

For starters, let's talk about sleep apnea, restless leg syndrome, periodic leg movement, narcolepsy. These sleep disorders, like insomnia, can leave you hanging on the ropes. While some are uncommon, they do occur, and often you'll become aware of them when you try to figure out what keeps you so sleepy during the day—why you're being robbed of sleep's benefits.

Sleep Apnea

Sleep apnea is the most common sleep disorder and reportedly affects 20 million adults. It increases markedly with age. (See Chapter 4: Sleep Changes with Aging.)

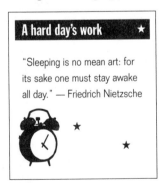

A hard day's work   ★

"Sleeping is no mean art: for its sake one must stay awake all day." — Friedrich Nietzsche

It's a condition that may cause you to stop breathing dozens or even hundreds of times a night during sleep. And each time is at least 10 seconds, sometimes up to a minute or two. The condition is predominantly found in men—some 30 times more likely than in premenopausal women. After menopause, the ratio is more even. Also, it is far more common in middle-aged and older men who are overweight. The clarion call of sleep apnea is explosively loud snoring.

Doesn't everyone snore now and then? Many people do, and benign snoring alone is no threat. The sleep apnea heralded by loud snoring can be life threatening, however. Occasional apnea is common and not significant. But pay attention if the sleeper with apnea has more than 10 or 20 episodes per hour or more than 100 per night. A heart condition is another cause for thorough checking, since the heart has difficulties functioning when oxygen pressure in the blood is below normal, as is often the case in obstructive sleep apnea.

How can you tell the snores of sleep apnea from plain old snoring? The telltale snoring is loud—earsplitting. Sleep partners say it's a sound like a jackhammer or a jet taking off. Often, next door neighbors can hear it. After not breathing for some seconds, the apneic sleeper sometimes resumes breathing with a loud explosive gasp. The pattern in sleep apnea is snoring interrupted by pauses, then gasps, then breathless periods, and so on. That kind of sleep, with some apneic sleepers not breathing for up to three-fourths of their sleep time, leaves some people more likely to have car accidents, disrupted work, troubles concentrating, irritability, anxiety, depression. And often without knowing why.

Sleep apnea does not suddenly occur, full-blown. As with most sleep disorders, it begins unobtrusively and worsens over time if nothing is done. So often, the victim of sleep apnea in its later forms is the last to know what's happening. He may notice waking frequently, thrashing about, gasping for air. He may notice morning headaches and tiredness during

---

Meditate on this ★

Combining meditation with other sleep-inducing strategies (such as going to bed drowsy and getting up at the same time) may help you fall asleep faster. When taught how to meditate and relax, insomniacs showed a 77 percent reduction in the time it took to fall asleep. Those whose treatment included only the tricks fell asleep 63 percent faster.

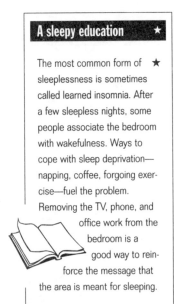

the day. But the snoring, gasping performance may elude him, happening as it
does during sleep. This obstructive sleep
apnea is caused by partial obstruction of
the airway. Muscles at the base of the
tongue relax, the uvula (the dingus
hanging down at the back of your
throat) often is enlarged and sagging,
throat muscles relax more than normal.
All of this is compounded in people who
are overweight. And the supine position
in sleep apparently fosters greater collapse. At times, the airway collapses,
breathing stops, snoring cuts off sometimes in mid-snore. Pressure to resume
breathing starts from the chest muscles
and nervous system, leading to resump-
tion, sometimes with a deep gasp.

What to do? See your doctor and explain what you can. It's helpful in
most cases to have your bed partner along (who probably will know the
sleep apnea better than the victim and will be anxious to help clear it
up.) Meanwhile, be overly cautious about alcohol, sleeping pills, and
tranquilizers at bedtime, since they all tend to further reduce muscle
tone. Avoid sleeping on your back, raise the head of your bed, or sleep
in an inclined chair. One homely and effective maneuver: Sew two tennis balls in a sock and attach the sock to the back of your pajama top.
(And you thought this was going to be easy?) Rolling onto the sock of
tennis balls a few times in your sleep will teach you to keep off your
back all night.

Some sleep specialists feel that much sleep apnea goes undiagnosed. If
you suspect that you have it, they advise seeing your doctor and consider getting an evaluation at a sleep disorders clinic.

Once diagnosed, the condition often responds to continuous positive
airway pressure, involving a nasal mask supplying constant air pressure

as you sleep. Surgery sometimes is indicated—a uvulopalatopharyngo-plasty, which is enough to cause apnea just pronouncing it—to recon-struct the airway. Sometimes having your tonsils or adenoids removed is recommended. Far less drastic is a treatment program that includes seri-ous weight reduction and avoidance of muscle relaxants.

What we have described is obstructive sleep apnea, the more serious and more common type. In central sleep apnea syndrome, the airway may stay open, but the diaphragm and chest muscles may stop working. Falling oxygen levels signal the brain to get the patient awake and breathing. This type of apnea is more likely in elderly patients with congestive heart failure or in neurological disorders.

Periodic Leg Movement

These are bouts of jerking and twitching during sleep. Each twitch may last about a second or two, and the episodes of movement happen about 10 to 60 seconds apart. Bouts of twitching may last a few minutes to several hours. Between bouts, a person may have sound sleep. Although uncommon, this condition is more likely with age, and perhaps one in three people over age 65 has at least mild periodic leg movement. The result often is excessive daytime sleepiness.

The cause is unknown, but specialists reassure us that it's not important medically. In other words, periodic leg movement may wake you and cause some lost sleep, but not cause permanent harm otherwise. Sometimes the movements seem to be medication-related—either intro-duction or withdrawal of a drug—but most are unresolved. The move-ments are not the same as whole body jerks as you're falling asleep; we all have those from time to time, and they are benign.

If you feel you have periodic leg movement disorder, see your doctor and prepare for a possible work-up at a sleep disorders center.

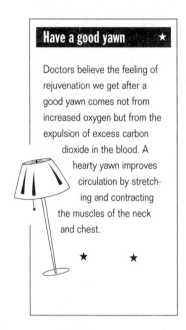

Have a good yawn ★

Doctors believe the feeling of rejuvenation we get after a good yawn comes not from increased oxygen but from the expulsion of excess carbon dioxide in the blood. A hearty yawn improves circulation by stretching and contracting the muscles of the neck and chest.

★   ★

Restless Leg Syndrome

The two conditions—periodic leg movement and restless leg syndrome—often occur in the same people. There are important differences. Restless leg syndrome usually interferes with falling asleep. It is a problem occurring during wake, not sleep.

And the feeling is deep in the muscles of the legs, an urge to move them. The sensation has been described as "worms crawling under the skin" or "crawling flesh," most often in the calves, but occasionally in the feet and thighs. Not a pretty simile, but there's nothing pleasant about this condition.

People who have it feel an almost uncontrollable urge to move, to get up and walk off the nervous feeling in the legs. While the sensation is not that of pain, it is uncomfortable enough to deprive a person of the ability to fall asleep. While the cause of restless leg syndrome has not been pinpointed, it seems to occur often in people who do not get sufficient exercise. If you have the condition, see your doctor, eliminate stimulants, and exercise your legs—walking seems to aid some afflicted people. Certain medications seem to help. For complete diagnosis, you may require a work-up at a sleep disorder clinic.

Narcolepsy

This is the one many sleep researchers love to study. It's the quintessential sleep disorder. If you are one of the few people with the condition, you'll be glad for any help the specialists can offer. Narcolepsy leaves the person totally frustrated. No amount of sleep seems to satisfy the need for more. And that need, for persons with narcolepsy, comes on abruptly and under almost any condition. Sudden sleep can take over during a meeting, while talking on the telephone, at a dinner party, while making love in extreme cases (which surely tests the strength of that relationship), and even while driving a car. Most narcoleptics recognize a brief warning of sleepiness, which gives the driver time to pull off the road, and the lover to make whatever magical explanation he or she comes up with.

Sleep specialists are learning more about narcolepsy each year, and this strange malady is much better understood now. It was thought to be quite rare. Today, it may afflict 1 in 1,000 people—still rare but less so than previous estimates.

Narcolepsy, because of its unique combination of symptoms, is reasonably simple to diagnose, although this needs to be done in a sleep disorders clinic or with a sleep specialist consultation.

Here's the condition: If you have narcolepsy or have had narcoleptic bouts, you won't forget them. As with other sleep disorders, it develops gradually.

At its peak presentation, classic narcolepsy is not only the sleep attack, but a triad of other symptoms: cataplexy, sleep paralysis, hypnogogic hallucinations. The sleep attack lasts from a few seconds to 20 to 30 minutes and happens most often during monotonous activity such as a lecture, concert, television viewing. It is an offshoot of REM sleep, but during the day. Cataplexy is bilateral loss of muscle control, anything from a slight buckling of the knees to sinking to the floor, for instance. Most cataplectic attacks are associated with periods of high emotion, primarily happy or joyful, not frightening or discouraging. Hypnogogic hallucinations are vivid dreamlike images, anxiety-producing, as the person drifts off to sleep or gradually wakes up. Sleep paralysis may occur also on awakening or going to sleep—a brief inability to move or speak for a moment or two while in transition.

At night, a narcoleptic falls asleep in a peculiar way that is consistent with the condition. He drops almost directly into REM sleep, without the long, normal initial period of non-REM. Also, there seems to be a strong genetic link; up to 50 percent of patients with narcolepsy may have an affected first-degree relative, some reports suggest.

All the signs and symptoms may not be present, but in classic narcolepsy, they are—the abrupt falling asleep, the cataplexy, the sleep paralysis, the hallucinations. People who have had such attacks do not forget them, and some even try to keep a lid on their emotions to prevent another cataplectic attack.

Treatment of narcolepsy is tricky and is often done through a sleep specialist. The condition usually begins before age 30, and can continue through old age. Stimulant medicine may help. Proper medications nearly always help with hypnogogic hallucinations and sleep paralysis. Carefully spaced naps may help. This curious condition needs to be handled through specialists who will design the treatment for the individual patient's needs.

Parasomnias

These are tangential conditions that take place during sleep, often during a special stage of sleep. They may be inherited. If your parent or uncle or aunt sleepwalked, you have an above average chance of doing it. (For an eye-opening look at sleepwalking and assorted mysteries in the night, read "The Night the Bed Fell," in *A Thurber Carnival*, by James Thurber. Thurber was not only one of our finest humorists, he was a flaming insomniac.)

Sleepwalking—

Also known as somnambulism, this is a disruption of delta sleep.

The person with sleepwalking tendencies may get up, walk around the house, even outside, even doing things like washing dishes, albeit clumsily. Children are prone to this; at least 15 percent of all children ages 5 to 12 sleepwalk at least once. And some 1 percent of adults walk in their sleep, probably responding to stress or emotions. (It can be a part of post-traumatic stress syndrome.) The walks last less than 10 minutes. If you've observed this, you know that the person has eyes open but is not seeing, or not recognizing. The next morning, the nighttime walks are seldom remembered. Treatment is benign, keeping the person out of danger (hiding the car keys, keeping doors and windows locked). Medication may be used in problem situations.

Sleep Terrors—

Another disorder of delta sleep, and sleepwalkers are prone to it.

This severe reaction can be frightening, to those who observe as well as those having the attack. Sleep terrors usually happen in the first hour or so of sleep and begin with a loud cry or scream, followed by intense, frenzied activity, with the person often thinking he or she is being chased. The attack may last 5 to 10 minutes, with heart palpatations, sweating, other signs of fear. Then the person is confused, but usually drops into sleep without much problem. Recollection on awakening is fuzzy or nonexistent.

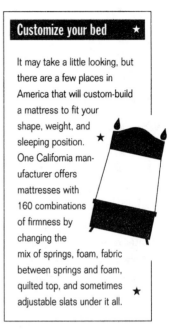

Customize your bed ★

It may take a little looking, but there are a few places in America that will custom-build a mattress to fit your shape, weight, and sleeping position. ★ One California manufacturer offers mattresses with 160 combinations of firmness by changing the mix of springs, foam, fabric between springs and foam, quilted top, and sometimes adjustable slats under it all. ★

Nightmares—

Related to REM sleep, dreams powerful enough to wake you up and you remember details, are nightmares. They are thought to be anxiety-related. We all have them and half of us have at least one a year. They are said to happen more often in creative types. (I report that without comment.) Common themes are falling, being chased, life-threatening situations. And themes do recur in your nightmares. (I have one about writing a sleep book, wherein...but no, no details.)

Sleep Talking—

This happens during REM sleep, when the large muscle groups are semi-paralyzed, but certain people can use their speech muscles to verbalize their dreams.

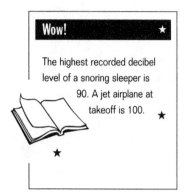

Wow! ★

The highest recorded decibel level of a snoring sleeper is 90. A jet airplane at takeoff is 100. ★

★

Some people who talk in their sleep can understand what you say to them. When they relax and fall back asleep, the next morning they rarely recall talking, which may be nature's way of forestalling marital discord.

Night Eating—

Also called the "Dagwood syndrome," this condition is not completely understood, but stems from a variety of causes. It happens more often in people who also have other sleep problems such as sleep walking, it may be caused by something as simple as poor or restricted diet during the day, it may be affected by medications prescribed for depression or other sleep disorders, and more.

With night eating, a person will waken during the night and have an uncontrollable urge to eat—an urge so strong that it's nearly impossible for him or her to get back to sleep without food. Some of this is a result of habit, of giving in to the urge and eating, even providing snacks for others, including children, who then come to expect it. Two-thirds of people with night eating problems are women, the condition usually first appears in the late 20s, and it is very rare for the condition to be connected to daytime eating problems.

It's important to try to break the habit, because it may result in excessive weight gain, possible choking while eating, potential injury in preparing foods—burns, cuts, and the like. And of course disrupted sleep. Try eating a protein-rich snack before retiring, drink water when you awake, and so on. It may be a conditioned reaction, so gradually try to change your habit. Check with your doctor to see if part of your problem may be medical, such as low blood sugar.

Further Reading

Of the many books about sleep, I recommend the following if you want more detail. They are written by recognized authorities in the field and are very readable (a happy and uncommon combination).

—Richard Graber

The Sleep Book: Understanding and Preventing Sleep Problems in People Over 50. Ernest Hartmann, M.D., An AARP Book, 1987; Scott Foresman and Company, Glenview, IL.

No More Sleepless Nights. Peter Hauri, Ph.D., and Shirley Linde, Ph.D., 1990; John Wiley & Sons, New York, NY.

Sleep Right in Five Nights: A Clear and Effective Guide for Conquering Insomnia. James Perl, Ph.D., 1993; W. Morrow, New York, NY.

Overcoming Insomnia: A Medical Program for Problem Sleepers. Donald R. Sweeney, M.D., Ph.D., 1989; The PIA Press, Bantam Doubleday Dell Publishing Group, Inc., New York, NY.

Appendix

Sleep Centers & Laboratories

Following is a listing of American Sleep Disorders Association Accredited Member Centers and Laboratories. Accredited Member Sleep Disorders Centers provide the diagnosis and treatment of all types of sleep related disorders. Accredited Member Laboratories specialize only in sleep related breathing disorders. You can obtain a current listing and additional information from the National Sleep Foundation, 1367 Connecticut Avenue NW, Suite 200, Washington, DC 20036.

ALABAMA

Brookwood Sleep Disorders Center
Brookwood Medical Center
2010 Brookwood Medical Center Drive
Birmingham, AL 35209
205-877-2486

Sleep Disorders Center of Alabama, Inc.
790 Montclair Road
Suite 200
Birmingham, AL 35213
205-599-1020

Sleep-Wake Disorders Center
University of Alabama at Birmingham
1713 6th Avenue South
CPM Building, Room 270
Birmingham, AL 35233-0018
205-934-7110

Sleep-Wake Disorders Center
Flowers Hospital
4370 West Main Street
P.O. Box 6907
Dothan, AL 36302
205-793-5000 x 1685

Alabama North Regional Sleep Disorders Center
250 Chateau Drive
Suite 235
Huntsville, AL 35801
205-880-6451

Huntsville Hospital Sleep Disorders Center
101 Sivley Road
Huntsville, AL 35801
205-517-8553

Sleep Disorders Center
Mobile Infirmary Medical Center
P.O. Box 2144
Mobile, AL 36652
334-431-5559

Southeast Regional Center for Sleep/Wake Disorders
Springhill Memorial Hospital
3719 Dauphin Street
Mobile, AL 36608
334-460-5319

USA Knollwood Sleep Disorders Center
University of South Alabama
Knollwood Park Hospital
5600 Girby Road
Mobile, AL 36693-3398
334-660-5757

Baptist Sleep Disorders Center
Baptist Medical Center
2105 East South Boulevard
Montgomery, AL 36116-2498
334-286-3252

Tuscaloosa Clinic Sleep Lab*
701 University Boulevard East
Tuscaloosa, AL 35401
205-349-4043

ALASKA

Sleep Disorders Center
Providence Alaska Medical Center
3200 Providence Drive
P.O. Box 196604
Anchorage, AK 99519-6604
907-261-3650

ARIZONA

Desert Samaritan Sleep Disorders Center
Desert Samaritan Medical Center
1400 South Dobson Road
Mesa, AZ 85202
602-835-3620

Samaritan Regional Sleep Disorders Program
Good Samaritan Regional Medical Center
1111 East McDowell Road
Phoenix, AZ 85006
602-239-5815

Sleep Disorders Center at Scottsdale Memorial Hospital
Scottsdale Memorial Hospital-North
10450 North 92nd Street
Scottsdale, AZ 85261-9930
602-860-3200

* Accredited as Specialty Laboratory for Sleep Related Breathing Disorders
All other programs are accredited full service Sleep Disorders Centers

Sleep Disorders Center
University of Arizona
1501 North Campbell Avenue
Tucson, AZ 85724
520-694-6112

ARKANSAS

Sleep Disorders Center
Washington Regional Medical Center
1125 North College
Fayetteville, AR 72703
501-442-1272

Pediatric Sleep Disorders
Arkansas Children's Hospital
800 Marshall Street
Little Rock, AR 72202-3591
501-320-1893

Sleep Disorders Center
Baptist Medical Center
9601 I-630, Exit 7
Little Rock, AR 72205-7299
501-227-1902

CALIFORNIA

WestMed Sleep Disorders Center
1101 South Anaheim Boulevard
Anaheim, CA 92805
714-491-1159

Mercy Sleep Laboratory*
Mercy San Juan Hospital
6501 Coyle Avenue
Carmichael, CA 95608
916-966-5552

Downey Comunity Hospital Sleep Disorders Center
Rio Hondo Foundation Hospital
8300 East Telegraph Road
Downey, CA 90240
310-806-6523

Palomar Medical Center Sleep Disorders Lab*
Palomar Medical Center
555 East Valley Parkway
Escondido, CA 95025
619-739-3457

Sleep Disorders Institute
St. Jude Medical Center
100 East Valencia Mesa Drive
Suite 308
Fullerton, CA 92635
714-992-3981

Glendale Adventist Medical Center Sleep Disorders Center
Glendale Adventist Medical Center
1509 Wilson Terrace
Glendale, CA 91206
818-409-8323

Sleep Disorders Center
Scripps Clinic and Research Foundation
10666 North Torrey Pines Road
La Jolla, CA 92037
619-554-8087

* Accredited as Specialty Laboratory for Sleep Related Breathing Disorders
All other programs are accredited full service Sleep Disorders Centers

Sleep Disorders Center
Grossmont District Hospital
P.O. Box 158
La Mesa, CA 92044-0300
619-644-4488

Memorial Sleep Disorders Center
Long Beach Memorial Medical Center
2801 Atlantic Avenue
P.O. Box 1428
Long Beach, CA 90801-1428
310-933-2091 or 310-426-1816

Sleep Disorders Center
Cedars-Sinai Medical Center
8700 Beverly Boulevard
Los Angeles, CA 90048-1869
310-855-2405

UCLA Sleep Disorders Center
710 Westwood Plaza
Los Angeles, CA 90095
310-206-8005

Sleep Disorders Center
Hoag Memorial Hospital Presbyterian
301 Newport Boulevard
P.O. Box 6100
Newport Beach, CA 92658-6100
714-760-2070

Sleep Evaluation Center
Northridge Hospital Medical Center
18300 Roscoe Boulevard
Northridge, CA 91328
818-885-5344

California Center for Sleep Disorders
3012 Summit Street
5th Floor, South Building
Oakland, CA 94609
510-834-8333

St. Joseph Hospital Sleep Disorders Center
1310 West Stewart Drive
Suite 403
Orange, CA 92668
714-771-8950

Sleep Disorders Center
UC Irvine Medical Center
101 City Drive South
Orange, CA 92668
714-456-5105

Sleep Disorders Center
Huntington Memorial Hospital
100 West California Boulevard
P.O. Box 7013
Pasadena, CA 91109-7013
818-397-3061

Sleep Disorders Center
Doctors Hospital - Pinole
2151 Appian Way
Pinole, CA 94564-2578
510-741-2525 and 800-640-9440

Pomona Valley Hospital Medical Center
Sleep Disorders Center
1798 North Garey Avenue
Pomona, CA 91767
909-865-9587

Sleep Disorders Center
Sequoia Hospital
170 Alameda de las Pulgas
Redwood City, CA 94062-2799
415-367-5137

Sleep Disorders Center at Riverside
Riverside Community Hospital
4445 Magnolia, E1
Riverside, CA 92501
909-788-3377

Sutter Sleep Disorders Center
650 Howe Avenue
Suite 910
Sacramento, CA 95825
916-646-3300

Mercy Sleep Disorders Center
Mercy Health Care San Diego
4077 Fifth Avenue
San Diego, CA 92103-2180
619-260-7378

San Diego Sleep Disorders Center
1842 Third Avenue
San Diego, CA 92101
619-235-0248

Sleep Disorders Center
California Pacific Medical Center
2340 Clay Street
Suite 237
San Francisco, CA 94155
415-923-3584

Sleep Disorders Center
San Jose Medical Center
675 East Santa Clara Street
San Jose, CA 95112
408-993-7005

The Sleep Disorders Center of Santa Barbara
2410 Fletcher Avenue
Suite 201
Santa Barbara, CA 93105
805-898-8845

Sleep Disorders Clinic
Stanford University
401 Quarry Road
Stanford, CA 94305
415-723-6601

Southern California Sleep Apnea Center*
Lombard Medical Group
2230 Lynn Road
Thousand Oaks, CA 91360
805-495-1066

Torrance Memorial Medical Center
Sleep Disorders Center
3330 West Lomita Boulevard
Torrance, CA 90505
310-517-4617

Sleep Disorders Laboratory*
Kaweah Delta District Hospital
400 West Mineral King Avenue
Visalia, CA 93291
209-625-7338

* Accredited as Specialty Laboratory for Sleep Related Breathing Disorders
All other programs are accredited full service Sleep Disorders Centers

West Hills Sleep Disorders Center
23101 Sherman Place
Suite 108
West Hills, CA 91307
818-715-0096

COLORADO

National Jewish/University of Colorado Sleep Center
1400 Jackson Street, A200
Denver, CO 80206
303-398-1523

Sleep Disorders Center
Presbyterian/St. Luke's Medical Center
1719 East 19th Avenue
Denver, CO 80218
303-839-6447

CONNECTICUT

New Haven Sleep Disorders Center
100 York Street, University Towers
New Haven, CT 06511
203-776-9578

Gaylord-Yale Sleep Laboratory*
Gaylord Hospital
Gaylord Farms Road
Wallingford, CT 06492
203-284-2853 or 203-284-2800 x 3355

---

* Accredited as Specialty Laboratory for Sleep Related Breathing Disorders
All other programs are accredited full service Sleep Disorders Centers

DELAWARE

No Accredited Members

DISTRICT OF COLUMBIA

Sleep Disorders Center
Georgetown University Hospital
3800 Reservoir Road Northwest
Washington, DC 20007-2197
202-784-3610

Sibley Memorial Hospital Sleep Disorders Center
5255 Loughboro Road Northwest
Washington DC 20016
202-364-7676

FLORIDA

Boca Raton Sleep Disorders Center
899 Meadows Road
Suite 101
Boca Raton, FL 33486
407-750-9881

Sleep Disorder Laboratory*
Broward General Medical Center
1600 South Andrews Avenue
Fort Lauderdale, FL 33316
305-355-5534

Center for Sleep Disordered Breathing*
P.O. Box 2982
Jacksonville, FL 32203
904-387-7300 x 8743

* Accredited as Specialty Laboratory for Sleep Related Breathing Disorders
All other programs are accredited full service Sleep Disorders Centers

Mayo Sleep Disorders Center
Mayo Clinic Jacksonville
4500 San Pablo Road
Jacksonville, FL 32224
904-953-7287

Watson Clinic Sleep Disorders Center
The Watson Clinic
1600 Lakeland Hills Boulevard
P.O. Box 95000
Lakeland, FL 33804-5000
813-680-7627

Atlantic Sleep Disorders Center
1401 South Apollo Boulevard
Melbourne, FL 32901
407-952-5191

Sleep Disorders Center
Mt. Sinai Medical Center
4300 Alton Road
Miami Beach, FL 33140
305-674-2613

Sleep Disorders Center
Miami Children's Hospital
6125 Southwest 31st Street
Miami, FL 33155
305-662-8330

University of Miami School of Medicine
JMH and VA Medical Center Sleep Disorders Center
Department of Neurology (D4-5)
P.O. Box 016960
Miami, FL 33101
305-324-3371

Florida Hospital Sleep Disorders Center
601 East Rollins Avenue
Orlando, FL 32803
407-897-1558

Holmes Sleep Disorders Center
Palm Bay Community Hospital
1425 Malabar Road Northeast
Suite 255
Palm Bay, FL 32907
407-728-5387

Sleep Disorders Center
Sarasota Memorial Hospital
1700 South Tamiami Trail
Sarasota, FL 34239
941-917-2525

St. Petersburg Sleep Disorders Center
2525 Pasadena Avenue South
Suite S
St. Petersburg, FL 33707
813-360-0853 or 800-242-3244 (in Florida)

Laboratory for Sleep Related Breathing Disorders*
University Community Hospital
3100 East Fletcher Avenue
Tampa, FL 33613
813-971-6000 x 7410

* Accredited as Specialty Laboratory for Sleep Related Breathing Disorders
All other programs are accredited full service Sleep Disorders Centers

GEORGIA

Atlanta Center for Sleep Disroders
303 Parkway
Box 44
Atlanta, GA 30312
404-265-3722

Sleep Disorders Center
Northside Hospital
1000 Johnson Ferry Road
Atlanta, GA 30342
404-851-9135

Sleep Disorders Center of Georgia
5505 Peachtree Dunwoody Road
Suite 370
Atlanta, GA 30342
404-257-0080

Promina Kennestone Sleep Disorders Center
Promina Kennestone Hospital
677 Church Street
Marietta, GA 30060
770-793-5353

Department of Sleep Disorders Medicine
Candler Hospital
5353 Reynolds Street
Savannah, GA 31405
912-692-6531

Sleep Disorders Center
Memorial Medical Center, Inc.
4700 Waters Avenue
Savannah, GA 31403
912-350-8327

Savannah Sleep Disorders Center
Saint Joseph's Hospital
#6 St. Joseph's Professional Plaza
11706 Mercy Boulevard
Savannah, GA 31419
912-927-5141

HAWAII

Pulmonary Sleep Disorders Center*
Kuakini Medical Center
347 North Kaukini Street
Honolulu, HI 96817
808-547-9119

Sleep Disorders Center of the Pacific
Straub Clinic & Hospital
888 South King Street
Honolulu, HI 96813
808-522-4448

IDAHO

No Accredited Members

ILLINOIS

Neurological Testing Center's Sleep Disorders Center
Northwestern Memorial Hospital
303 East Superior, Passavant 1044
Chicago, IL 60611
312-908-8120

* Accredited as Specialty Laboratory for Sleep Related Breathing Disorders
All other programs are accredited full service Sleep Disorders Centers

Sleep Disorder Service and Research Center
Rush-Presbyterian-St. Luke's
1653 West Congress Parkway
Chicago, IL 60612
312-942-5440

Sleep Disorders Center
The University of Chicago Hospitals
5841 South Maryland, MC2091
Chicago, IL 60637
312-702-1782

Sleep Disorders Center
Evanston Hospital
2650 Ridge Avenue
Evanston, IL 60201
708-570-2567

C. Duane Morgan Sleep Disorders Center
Methodist Medical Center of Illinois
221 Northeast Glen Oak Avenue
Peoria, IL 61636
309-672-4966

SIU School of Medicine
Memorial Medical Center Sleep Disorders Center
Memorial Medical Center
800 North Rutledge
Springfield, IL 62781
217-788-4269

Carle Regional Sleep Disorders Center
611 West Park Street
Urbana, IL 61801-2595
217-383-3364

INDIANA

St. Mary's Sleep Disorders Center*
St. Mary's Medical Center
3700 Washington Avenue
Evansville, IN 47750
812-479-4960

St. Joseph Sleep Disorders Center
St. Joseph Medical Center
700 Broadway
Fort Wayne, IN 46802
219-425-3552

Sleep/Wake Disorders Center
Community Hospitals of Indianapolis
1500 North Ritter Avenue
Indianapolis, IN 46219
317-355-4275

Sleep Disorders Center
Winona Memorial Hospital
3232 North Meridian Street
Indianapolis, IN 46208
317-927-2100

Sleep Alertness Center
Lafayette Home Hospital
2400 South Street
Lafayette, IN 47904
317-447-6811 x 2840

Sleep Disorders Center
Good Samaritan Hospital
520 South 7th Street
Vincennes, IN 47591
812-885-3877

* Accredited as Specialty Laboratory for Sleep Related Breathing Disorders
All other programs are accredited full service Sleep Disorders Centers

IOWA

Sleep Disorders Center
Genesis Medical Center
1401 West Central Park
Davenport, IA 52804
319-383-1966

Sleep Disorders Center
The Department of Neurology
The University of Iowa Hospitals and Clinics
Iowa City, IA 52242
319-356-3813

KANSAS

Sleep Disorders Center
St. Francis Hospital and Medical Center
1700 Southwest 7th Street
Topeka, KS 66606-1690
913-295-7900

Sleep Disorders Center
Wesley Medical Center
550 North Hillside
Wichita, KS 67214-4976
316-688-2663

KENTUCKY

Sleep Diagnostics Lab*
Greenview Regional Medical Center
1801 Ashley Circle
Bowling Green, KY 42101
502-793-2172

* Accredited as Specialty Laboratory for Sleep Related Breathing Disorders
All other programs are accredited full service Sleep Disorders Centers

Sleep Lab*
The Medical Center at Bowling Green
250 Park Street
P.O. Box 90010
Bowling Green, KY 42101-9010
502-745-1024

The Sleep Disorder Center of St. Luke Hospital
St. Luke Hospital, Inc.
85 North Grand Avenue
Fort Thomas, KY 41075
606-572-3535

Sleep Disorders Center
St. Joseph's Hospital
One St. Joseph Drive
Lexington, KY 40504
606-278-0444

Sleep Apnea Center*
Good Samaritan Hospital
310 South Limestone
Lexington, KY 40508
606-252-6612 x 7331

Sleep Disorders Center
Audubon Regional Medical Center
One Audubon Plaza Drive
Louisville, KY 40217
502-636-7459

Sleep Disorders Center
University of Louisville Hospital
530 South Jackson Street
Louisville, KY 40202
502-562-3792

* Accredited as Specialty Laboratory for Sleep Related Breathing Disorders
All other programs are accredited full service Sleep Disorders Centers

Regional Medical Center Lab for Sleep-Related Breathing Disorders*
900 Hospital Drive
Madisonville, KY 42431
502-825-5918

LOUISIANA

Mercy + Baptist Sleep Disorders Center
Tenetsub, Inc.
2700 Napoleon Avenue
New Orleans, LA 70115
504-896-5439

Tulane Sleep Disorders Center
1415 Tulane Avenue
New Orleans, LA 70112
504-588-5231

The Neurology and Sleep Clinic
2205 East 70th Street
Shreveport, LA 71105
318-797-1585

LSU Sleep Disorders Center
Louisiana State University Medical Center
P.O. Box 33932
Shreveport, LA 71130-3932
318-675-5365

MAINE

Sleep Laboratory*
Maine Medical Center
22 Bramhall Street
Portland, ME 04102
207-871-2279

* Accredited as Specialty Laboratory for Sleep Related Breathing Disorders
All other programs are accredited full service Sleep Disorders Centers

MARYLAND

The Johns Hopkins Sleep Disorders Center
Asthma and Allergy Building
Room 4B50
Johns Hopkins Bayview Medical Center
5501 Hopkins Bayview Circle
Baltimore, MD 21224
410-550-0571

Maryland Sleep Disorders Center, Inc.
Ruxton Towers, Suite 211
8415 Bellona Lane
Baltimore, MD 21204
410-494-9773

Shady Grove Sleep Disorders Center
14915 Broschart Road
Suite 102
Rockville, MD 20850
301-251-5905

MASSACHUSETTS

Sleep Disorders Center
Beth Israel Hospital
330 Brookline Avenue, KS430
Boston, MA 02215
617-667-3237

Sleep Disorders Center
Lahey-Hitchcock Clinic
41 Mall Road
Burlington, MA 01805
617-273-8251

Sleep Disorders Institute of Central New England
Saint Vincent Hospital
25 Winthrop Street
Worcester, MA 01604
508-798-6212

MICHIGAN

Sleep/Wake Disorders Laboratory (127B)
VA Medical Center
Southfield & Outer Drive
Allen Park, MI 48101
313-562-6000 x 3663 or 3662

Sleep Disorders Center
St. Joseph Mercy Hospital
P.O. Box 995
Ann Arbor, MI 48106
313-712-4651

Sleep Disorders Center
University of Michigan Hospitals
1500 East Medical Center Drive
Med Inn C433, Box 0842
Ann Arbor, MI 48109-0115
313-936-9068

Sleep Disorders Clinic
Bay Medical Center
1900 Columbus Avenue
Bay City, MI 48708
517-894-3332

Sleep Disorders Center
Henry Ford Hospital
2921 West Grand Boulevard
Detroit, MI 48202
313-972-1800

Sleep Disorders Center
Butterworth Hospital
100 Michigan Street Northeast
Grand Rapids, MI 49503
616-732-3759

Sleep Disorders Center
W.A. Foote Memorial Hospital, Inc.
205 North East Avenue
Jackson, MI 49201
517-788-4750

Borgess Sleep Disorders Center
Borgess Medical Center
1521 Gull Road
Kalamazoo, MI 49001
616-226-7081

Michigan Capital Healthcare Sleep/Wake Center
2025 South Washington Avenue
Suite 300
Lansing, MI 48910-0817
517-334-2510

Sparrow Sleep Center
Sparrow Hospital
1215 East Michigan Avenue
P.O. Box 30480
Lansing, MI 48909-7980

Sleep Disorders Center
Oakwood Downriver Medical Center
25750 West Outer Drive
Lincoln Park, MI 48146-1599
313-382-6165

Sleep & Respiratory Associates of Michigan
28200 Franklin Road
Southfield, MI 48034
810-350-2722

Munson Sleep Disorders Center
Munson Medical Center
1105 6th Street, MPB Suite 307
Traverse City, MI 49684-2386
800-358-9641 or 616-935-6600

Sleep Disorders Institute
44199 Dequindre, Suite 311
Troy, MI 48098
810-879-0707

MINNESOTA

Duluth Regional Sleep Disorders Center
St. Mary's Medical Center
407 East Third Street
Duluth, MN 55805
218-726-4692

Sleep Disorders Center
Abbott Northwestern Hospital
800 E. 28th Street at Chicago Avenue
Minneapolis, MN 55407
612-863-4516

Minnesota Regional Sleep Disorders Center, #867B
Hennepin County Medical Center
701 Park Avenue South
Minneapolis, MN 55415
612-347-6288

Mayo Sleep Disorders Center
Mayo Clinic
200 First Street Southwest
Rochester, MN 55905
507-266-8900

Sleep Disorders Center
Methodist Hospital
6500 Excelsior Boulevard
St. Louis Park, MN 55426
612-993-6083

St. Joseph's Sleep Diagnostic Center
St. Joseph's Hospital
69 West Exchange Street
St. Paul, MN 55102
612-232-3682

MISSISSIPPI

Sleep Disorders Center
Memorial Hospital at Gulfport
P.O. Box 1810
Gulfport, MS 39501
601-865-3152

Sleep Disorders Center
Forrest General Hospital
P.O. Box 16389

6051 Highway 49
Hattiesburg, MS 39404
601-288-4970 or 800-280-8520

Sleep Disorders Center
University of Mississippi Medical Center
2500 North State Street
Jackson, MS 39216-4505
601-984-4820

MISSOURI

Sleep Medicine and Research Center
St. Luke's Hospital
232 South Woods Mill Road
Chesterfield, MO 63017
314-851-6030

University of Missouri Sleep Disorders Center
M-741 Neurology
University Hospital and Clinics
One Hospital Drive
Columbia, MO 65212
314-884-SLEEP or 800-ADD-SLEEP

Sleep Disorders Center
Research Medical Center
2316 East Meyer Boulevard
Kansas City, MO 64132-1199
816-276-4334

Sleep Disorders Center
St. Luke's Hosptial
4400 Wornall Road
Kansas City, MO 64111
816-932-3207

Cox Regional Sleep Disorders Center
3800 South National Avenue
Suite LL 150
Springfield, MO 65807
417-269-5575

Sleep Disorders & Research Center
Deaconess Medical Center
6150 Oakland Avenue
St. Louis, MO 63139
314-768-3100

Sleep Disorders Center
St. Louis University Medical Center
1221 South Grand Boulevard
St. Louis, MO 63104
314-577-8705

MONTANA

No Accredited Members

NEBRASKA

Great Plains Regional Sleep Physiology Center
Lincoln General Hospital
2300 South 16th Street
Lincoln, NE 68502
402-473-5338

Sleep Disorders Center
Clarkson Hospital
4350 Dewey Avenue
Omaha, NE 68105-1018
402-552-2286

Sleep Disorders Center
Methodist/Richard Young Hospital
2566 St. Mary's Avenue
Omaha, NE 68105
402-536-6305

NEVADA

Regional Center for Sleep Disorders
Sunrise Hospital and Medical Center
3186 South Maryland Parkway
Las Vegas, NV 89109
702-731-8365

The Sleep Clinic of Nevada
1012 East Sahara Avenue
Las Vegas, NV 89104
702-893-0020

Washoe Sleep Disorders Center and Sleep Laboratory
Washoe Professional Building and Washoe Medical Center
75 Pringle Way, Suite 701
Reno, NV 89502
702-328-4700 or 702-328-4701

NEW HAMPSHIRE

Sleep-Wake Disorders Center
Hampstead Hospital
East Road
Hampstead, NH 03841
603-329-5311 x 240

Sleep Disorders Center
Dartmouth-Hitchcock Medical Center
One Medical Center Drive
Lebanon, NH 03756
603-650-7534

NEW JERSEY

Institute for Sleep/Wake Disorders
Hackensack Medical Center
385 Prospect Avenue
Hackensack, NJ 07601
201-996-2992

Sleep Disorder Center of Morristown Memorial Hospital
95 Mount Kemble Avenue
2nd Floor, Thebaud Building
Morristown, NJ 07962
201-971-4567

Comprehensive Sleep Disorders Center
Robert Wood Johnson University Hospital
UMDNJ-RWJ Medical School
One Robert Wood Johnson Place
P.O. Box 2601
New Brunswick, NJ 08903-2601
908-937-8683

Sleep Disorders Center
Newark Beth Israel Medical Center
201 Lyons Avenue
Newark, NJ 07112
201-926-7163

Mercer Medical Center Sleep Disorders Center
Mercer Medical Center
446 Bellevue Avenue
P.O. Box 1658
Trenton, NJ 08607
609-394-4167

NEW MEXICO

University Hospital Sleep Disorders Center
University of New Mexico Hospital
4775 Indian School Road Northeast
Suite 307
Albuquerque, NM 87110
505-272-6110

NEW YORK

Capital Region Sleep/Wake Disorders Center
St. Peter's Hospital and Albany Medical Center
25 Hackett Boulevard
Albany, NY 12208
518-436-9253

Sleep-Wake Disorders Center
Montefiore Medical Center
111 East 210th Street
Bronx, NY 10467
718-920-4841

St. Joseph's Hospital Sleep Disorders Center
St. Joseph's Hospital
555 East Market Street
Elmira, NY 14902
607-733-6541 x 7008

Sleep Disorders Center
Winthrop-University Hospital
222 Station Plaza North
Mineola, NY 11501
516-663-3907

Sleep-Wake Disorders Center
Long Island Jewish Medical Center
270-05 76th Avenue
New Hyde Park, NY 11042
718-470-7058

The Sleep Disorders Center
Columbia Presbyterian Medical Center
161 Fort Washington Avenue
New York, NY 10032
212-305-1860

Sleep Disorders Institute
St. Luke's/Roosevelt Hospital Center
Amsterdam Avenue at 114th Street
New York, NY 10025
212-523-1700

Sleep Disorders Center of Rochester
2110 Clinton Avenue South
Rochester, NY 14618
716-442-4141

Sleep Disorders Center
State University of New York at Stony Brook
University Hospital
MR 120A
Stony Brook, NY 11794-7139
516-444-2916

The Sleep Center
Community General Hospital
Broad Road
Syracuse, NY 13215
315-492-5877

The Sleep Laboratory*
945 East Genesee Street
Suite 300
Syracuse, NY 13210
315-475-3379

Sleep-Wake Disorders Center
New York Hospital-Cornell Medical Center
21 Bloomingdale Road
White Plains, NY 10605
914-997-5751

NORTH CAROLINA

Sleep Medicine Center of Asheville
1091 Hendersonville Road
Asheville, NC 28803
704-277-7533

---

* Accredited as Specialty Laboratory for Sleep Related Breathing Disorders
All other programs are accredited full service Sleep Disorders Centers

Sleep Center
University Hospital
P.O. Box 560727
Charlotte, NC 28256
704-548-6848

Sleep Disorders Center
The Moses H. Cone Memorial Hospital
1200 North Elm Street
Greensboro, NC 27401-1020
910-574-7406

Sleep Disorders Center
North Carolina Baptist Hospital
Bowman Gray School of Medicine
Medical Center Boulevard
Winston-Salem, NC 27157
910-716-5288

Summit Sleep Disorders Center
160 Charlois Boulevard
Winston-Salem, NC 27103
910-765-9431

NORTH DAKOTA

Sleep Disorders Center
MeritCare Hospital
720 4th Street North
Fargo, ND 58122
701-234-5673

OHIO

Sleep Disorders Center
Bethesda Oak Hospital
619 Oak Street
Cincinnati, OH 45206
513-569-6320

The Center for Research in Sleep Disorders
Affiliated with Mercy Hospital of Hamilton/Fairfield
1275 East Kemper Road
Cincinnati, OH 45246
513-671-3101

Sleep Disorders Center
The Cleveland Clinic Foundation
9500 Euclid Avenue, Desk S-83
Cleveland, OH 44195
216-444-8275

Sleep Disorders Center
Rainbow Babies Children's Hospital
Case Western Reserve University
11100 Euclid Avenue
Cleveland, OH 44106
216-844-1301

Sleep Disorders Center
The Ohio State University Medical Center
Rhodes Hall, S1032
410 West 10th Avenue
Columbus, OH 43210-1228
614-293-8296

The Center for Sleep & Wake Disorders
Miami Valley Hospital
One Wyoming Street
Suite G-200
Dayton, OH 45409
513-220-2515

Ohio Sleep Medicine Institute
4975 Bradenton Avenue
Dublin, OH 43017
614-766-0773

Sleep Disorders Center
Kettering Medical Center
3535 Southern Boulevard
Kettering, OH 45429-1295
513-296-7805

Sleep Disorders Center
St. Vincent Medical Center
2213 Cherry Street
Toledo, OH 43608-2691
419-321-4980

Northwest Ohio Sleep Disorders Center
The Toledo Hospital
Harris-McIntosh Tower, Second Floor
2142 North Cove Boulevard
Toledo, OH 43606
419-471-5629

Sleep Disorders Center
Good Samaritan Medical Center
800 Forest Avenue
Zanesville, OH 43701
614-454-5855

OKLAHOMA

Sleep Disorders Center of Oklahoma
Southwest Medical Center of Oklahoma
4401 South Western Avenue
Oklahoma City, OK 73109
405-636-7700

OREGON

Sleep Disorders Center
Sacred Heart Medical Center
1255 Hilyard Street
P.O. Box 10905
Eugene, OR 97440
503-686-7224

Sleep Disorders Center
Rogue Valley Medical Center
2825 East Barnett Road
Medford, OR 97504
503-770-4320

Pacific Northwest Sleep Disorders Program
1849 Northwest Kearney Street
Suite 202
Portland, OR 97210
503-228-4414

Sleep Disorders Laboratory*
Providence Medical Center
4805 Northeast Glisan Street
Portland, OR 97213
503-215-6552

* Accredited as Specialty Laboratory for Sleep Related Breathing Disorders
All other programs are accredited full service Sleep Disorders Centers

Salem Hospital Sleep Disorders Center
Salem Hospital
665 Winter Street Southeast
Salem, OR 97309-5014
503-370-5170

PENNSYLVANIA

Sleep Disorders Center
Abington Memorial Hospital
1200 Old York Road
2nd Floor Rorer Building
Abington, PA 19001
215-576-2226

Sleep Disorders Center
Lower Bucks Hospital
501 Bath Road
Bristol, PA 19007
215-785-9752

Sleep Disorders Center*
The Good Samaritan Medical Center
1020 Franklin Street
Johnstown, PA 15905
814-533-1661

Sleep Disorders Center of Lancaster
Lancaster General Hospital
555 North Duke Street
Lancaster, PA 17604-3555
717-290-5910

* Accredited as Specialty Laboratory for Sleep Related Breathing Disorders
All other programs are accredited full service Sleep Disorders Centers

Sleep Disorders Center
The Medical College of Pennsylvania
3200 Henry Avenue
Philadelphia, PA 19129
215-842-4250

Penn Center for Sleep Disorders
Hospital of the University of Pennsylvania
3400 Spruce Street, 11 Gates West
Philadelphia, PA 19104
215-662-7772

Sleep Disorders Center
Thomas Jefferson University
1025 Walnut Street
Suite 316
Philadelphia, PA 19107
215-955-6175

Pulmonary Sleep Evaluation Center*
University of Pittsburgh Medical Center
Montefiore University Hospital
3459 Fifth Avenue, S639
Pittsburgh, PA 15213
412-692-2880

Sleep and Chronobiology Center
Western Psychiatric Institute and Clinic
3811 O'Hara Street
Pittsburgh, PA 15213-2593
412-624-2246

* Accredited as Specialty Laboratory for Sleep Related Breathing Disorders
All other programs are accredited full service Sleep Disorders Centers

Sleep Disorders Center
Community Medical Center
1822 Mulberry Street
Scranton, PA 18510
717-969-8931

Sleep Disorders Center
Crozer-Chester Medical Center
One Medical Center Boulevard
Upland, PA 19013-3975
610-447-2689

Sleep Disorders Center
The Lankenau Hospital
100 Lancaster Avenue
Wynnewood, PA 19096
610-645-3400

RHODE ISLAND

Sleep Disorders Center
Rhode Island Hospital
593 Eddy Street, APC-301
Providence, RI 02903
401-444-4269

SOUTH CAROLINA

Roper Sleep/Wake Disorders Center
Roper Hospital
316 Calhoun Street
Charleston, SC 29401-1125
803-724-2246

Sleep Disorders Center of South Carolina
Baptist Medical Center
Taylor at Marion Streets
Columbia, SC 29220
803-771-5847

Sleep Disorders Center
Greenville Memorial Hospital
701 Grove Road
Greenville, SC 29605
803-455-8916

Children's Sleep Disorders Center*
Self Memorial Hospital
1325 Spring Street
Greenwood, SC 29646
803-227-4449 or 4489

Sleep Disorders Center
Spartanburg Regional Medical Center
101 East Wood Street
Spartanburg, SC 29303
803-560-6904

SOUTH DAKOTA

The Sleep Center
Rapid City Regional Hospital
353 Fairmont Boulevard
P.O. Box 6000
Rapid City, SD 57709
605-341-8037

* Accredited as Specialty Laboratory for Sleep Related Breathing Disorders
All other programs are accredited full service Sleep Disorders Centers

Sleep Disorders Center
Sioux Valley Hospital
1100 South Euclid
Sioux Falls, SD 57117-5039
605-333-6302

TENNESSEE

Sleep Disorders Laboratory*
Regional Hospital of Jackson
367 Hospital Boulevard
Jackson, TN 38303
901-661-2148

Sleep Disorders Cener
Ft. Sanders Regional Medical Center
1901 West Clinch Avenue
Knoxville, TN 37916
423-541-1375

Sleep Disorders Center
St. Mary's Medical Center
900 East Oak Hill Avenue
Knoxville, TN 37917-4556
423-545-6746

BMH Sleep Disorders Center
Baptist Memorial Hospital
899 Madison Avenue
Memphis, TN 38146
901-227-5337

Methodist Sleep Disorders Center
Methodist Hospital of Memphis
1265 Union Avenue (12 Thomas)
Memphis, TN 38104
901-726-7378

* Accredited as Specialty Laboratory for Sleep Related Breathing Disorders
All other programs are accredited full service Sleep Disorders Centers

Sleep Disorders Center
Centennial Medical Center
2300 Patterson Street
Nashville, TN 37203
615-342-1670

Sleep Disorders Center
Saint Thomas Hospital
P.O. Box 380
Nashville, TN 37202
615-222-2068

TEXAS

NWTH Sleep Disorders Center
Northwest Texas Hospital
P.O. Box 1110
Amarillo, TX 79175
806-354-1954

Sleep Disorders Center for Children
Children's Medical Center of Dallas
1935 Motor Street
Dallas, TX 75235
214-640-2793

Sleep Medicine Institute
Presbyterian Hospital of Dallas
8200 Walnut Hill Lane
Dallas, TX 75231
214-345-8563

Sleep Disorders Center
Columbia Medical Center West
1801 North Oregon
El Paso, TX 79902
915-521-1257

Sleep Disorders Center
Providence Memorial Hospital
2001 North Oregon
El Paso, TX 79902
915-577-6152

All Saints Sleep Disorders Diagnostic & Treatment Center
All Saints Episcopal Hospital
1400 8th Avenue
Fort Worth, TX 76104
817-927-6120

Sleep Disorders Center
Department of Psychiatry
Baylor College of Medicine and VA Medical Center
One Baylor Plaza
Houston, TX 77030
713-798-4886

Sleep Disorders Center
Spring Branch Medical Center
8850 Long Point Road
Suite 420 S
Houston, TX 77055
713-973-6483 or 713-794-7563

Sleep Disorders Center
Scott and White Clinic
2401 South 31st Street
Temple, TX 76508
817-724-2554

UTAH

Intermountain Sleep Disorders Center
LDS Hospital
325 8th Avenue
Salt Lake City, UT 84143
801-321-3617

University Health Sciences Center
Sleep Disorders Center
50 North Medical Drive
Salt Lake City, UT 84132
801-581-2016

VERMONT

No Accredited Members

VIRGINIA

Fairfax Sleep Disorders Center
3289 Woodburn Road
Suite 360
Annandale, VA 22003
703-876-9870

Sleep Disorders Center
Eastern Virginia Medical School
Sentara Norfolk General Hospital
600 Gresham Drive
Norfolk, VA 23507
804-668-3322

Sleep Disorders Center
Medical College of Virginia
P.O. Box 710-MCV
Richmond, VA 23298-0710
804-828-1490

Sleep Disorders Center
Community Hospital of Roanoke Valley
P.O. Box 12946
Roanoke, VA 24029
703-985-8526

WASHINGTON

Sleep Disorders Center for Southwest Washington
St. Peter Hospital
413 North Lilly Road
Olympia, WA 98506
206-493-7436

Richland Sleep Laboratory*
800 Swift Boulevard
Suite 260
Richland, WA 99352
509-946-4632

---

* Accredited as Specialty Laboratory for Sleep Related Breathing Disorders
All other programs are accredited full service Sleep Disorders Centers

Providence Sleep Disorders Center
Jefferson Tower
Suite 203
1600 East Jefferson
Seattle, WA 98122
206-320-2575

Seattle Sleep Disorders Center
Swedish Medical Center/Ballard
P.O. Box 70707
Seattle, WA 98107-1507
206-781-6359

Sleep Disorders Center
Sacred Heart Doctors Building
105 West Eighth Avenue
Suite 418
Spokane, WA 99204
509-455-4895

St. Clare Sleep Related Breathing Disorders Clinic*
St. Clare Hospital
11315 Bridgeport Way Southwest
Tacoma, WA 98499
206-581-6951

WEST VIRGINIA

Sleep Disorders Center
Charleston Area Medical Center
501 Morris Street - P.O. Box 1393
Charleston, WV 25325
304-348-7507

* Accredited as Specialty Laboratory for Sleep Related Breathing Disorders
All other programs are accredited full service Sleep Disorders Centers

WISCONSIN

Regional Sleep Disorders Center
Appleton Medical Center
1818 North Meade Street
Appleton, WI 54911
414-738-6460

Luther/Midelfort Sleep Disorders Center
Luther Hospital/Midelfort Clinic
1221 Whipple Street
P.O. Box 4105
Eau Claire, WI 54702-4105
715-838-3165

St. Vincent Hospital Sleep Disorders Center
St. Vincent Hospital
P.O. Box 13508
Green Bay, WI 54307-3508
414-431-3041

Wisconsin Sleep Disorders Center
Gundersen Clinic, Ltd.
1836 South Avenue
La Crosse, WI 54601
608-782-7300 x 2870

Comprehensive Sleep Disorders Center
B6/579 Clinical Science Center
University of Wisconsin Hospitals and Clinics
600 Highland Avenue
Madison, WI 53792
608-263-2387

Marshfield Sleep Disorders Center
Marshfield Clinic
1000 North Oak Avenue
Marshfield, WI 54449
715-387-5397

Milwaukee Regional Sleep Disorders Center
Columbia Hospital
2025 East Newport Avenue
Milwaukee, WI 53211
414-961-4650

St. Luke's Sleep Disorders Center
St. Luke's Medical Center
2900 West Oklahoma Avenue
Milwaukee, WI 53201-2901
414-649-6572

Sleep/Wake Disorders Center
St. Mary's Hospital
2320 North Lake Drive
P.O. Box 503
Milwaukee, WI 53201-4565
414-291-1275

WYOMING

No Accredited Members

Index